Renal
Pathophysiology
—the essentials

Renal Pathophysiology
—the essentials

Edited by

J. Gary Abuelo, M.D.

Associate Professor of Medicine
Brown University Program in Medicine
Associate Physician
Division of Renal Diseases
Rhode Island Hospital
Providence, Rhode Island

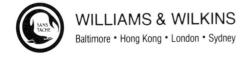

WILLIAMS & WILKINS
Baltimore • Hong Kong • London • Sydney

Editor: Timothy S. Satterfield
Associate Editor: Linda Napora
Copy Editor: Stephen Siegforth
Design: Bob Och
Illustration Planning: Wayne Hubbel
Production: Raymond E. Reter

Copyright © 1989
Williams & Wilkins
428 East Preston Street
Baltimore, Maryland 21202, USA

Accurate indications, adverse reactions, and dosage schedules for drugs are provided in this book, but it is possible that they may change. The reader is urged to review the package information data of the manufacturers of the medications mentioned.

Printed in the United States of America

Library of Congress Cataloging in Publication Data

Renal pathophysiology.

   Includes bibliographies and index.
   1. Kidneys—Pathophysiology.   I. Abuelo, J. Gary.
[DNLM: 1. Kidney Diseases—physiopathology.
WJ 300 R3923]
RC903.9.R48   1989   616.6'1   88-17115
ISBN 0-683-00050-0

89 90 91 92 93
1 2 3 4 5 6 7 8 9 10

Preface

The purpose of this book is to make life easier and more interesting for medical students trying to gain a working knowledge of renal pathophysiology in the few short weeks usually allotted to the subject in most medical schools. The authors have been teaching the renal pathophysiology course at the Program in Medicine of Brown University for several years and have been distributing lecture notes to the class in the form of a syllabus with the essential material of the course. Because this syllabus provides a concise and organized presentation of the subject, we decided to prepare it for publication. This short book is the result. Although it was primarily written for a second year course, the book can also be of use to medical students in their clinical years and serve as a reference source for pharmacology and nursing students as well as for nurses specializing in renal disease and dialysis.

In *Renal Pathophysiology—The Essentials* we consider pathophysiology from two viewpoints. First, it is a science that studies and explains the pathogenesis and manifestations of clinical disorders. It has a particularly important place in the preclinical years since it integrates information from physiology, biochemistry, anatomy, microbiology and pathology. Second, it interdigitates with pharmacology and physical diagnosis and naturally serves as an introduction to clinical medicine. To emphasize the applicability of renal pathophysiology to patient care, we have organized our book into the major renal and electrolyte disorders; we include for each condition a brief discussion of diagnosis and treatment and provide clinically oriented problems at the end of each chapter for the reader to solve.

Chapter 1 presents a review of normal renal and electrolyte physiology which the student presumably studied in his/her first year. Chapters 2 to 5 consider the principal fluid and electrolyte disturbances, i.e., volume, tonicity, acid-base and potassium disorders. Chapters 6 to 10 cover the pathophysiology of renal disease including glomerular, perfusion and urinary outflow disorders; stone formation; and acute and chronic renal failure. The final two chapters are on hypertension and the urinalysis. We have not included renal pathology, the pharmacology of diuretic and antihypertensive drugs or the disorders of calcium and phosphorus metabolism because they are normally taught in second year pathology, pharmacology and endocrinology courses, respectively.

Although the concise treatment that we give to our subject is advantageous to medical students as they learn patient care, this approach unfortunately cannot do justice to the fact that the fascinating science of renal pathophysiology is constantly evolving and is the focus of active research. Students interested in going beyond the practical version of the material provided here are encouraged to explore the Suggested Readings.

I gratefully acknowledge the assistance and contributions of the following people: Serafino Garella, who was the director of the renal pathophysiology course at Brown University for many years. He set high standards for course content, excellence in teaching, and above all, clarity in thinking that I hope characterizes this book. Nathana Lurvey, a medical student and a participant in the Rose Writing Fellow Program at Brown University, read and made helpful recommendations on the manuscript. Milton H. Lipsky, medical illustrator at the Rhode Island Hospital, did the line drawings and gave valuable advice during the preparation of the other illustrations. Charlene McGloin provided patience and skillful secretarial assistance.

Finally, a special acknowledgment is given Serafino Garella and Richard Solomon, portions of whose old syllabus sections form part of the framework of this book.

Contributors

J. Gary Abuelo, M.D. Associate Professor of Medicine, Brown University Program in Medicine; Associate Physician, Division of Renal Diseases, Rhode Island Hospital, Providence, Rhode Island

Andrew S. Brem, M.D. Assistant Professor of Pediatrics, Brown University Program in Medicine; Director, Division of Pediatric Nephrology, Rhode Island Hospital, Providence, Rhode Island

Jaime S. Carvalho, M.D. Department of Medicine, Veterans Administration Medical Center; Division of Biological and Medical Sciences, Brown University Program in Medicine, Providence, Rhode Island

Bruce S. Chang, M.D., F.A.C.P. Warwick, Rhode Island

David D. Clark, M.D. Clinical Assistant Professor of Medicine, Brown University Program in Medicine; Associate Physician, Division of Renal Diseases, Rhode Island Hospital, Providence, Rhode Island

Sewell I. Kahn, M.D. Clinical Assistant Professor of Medicine, Brown University Program in Medicine, Providence, Rhode Island; Medical Director, Rhode Island Renal Institute, Warwick, Rhode Island

Rex L. Mahnensmith, M.D. Assistant Professor of Medicine, Brown University Program in Medicine; Director, Division of Nephrology, The Miriam Hospital, Providence, Rhode Island

Pavel Vancura, M.D. Clinical Assistant Professor of Medicine, Brown University Program in Medicine, Providence, Rhode Island

Thasia G. Woodworth, M.D. Director of Clinical Affairs, Seragen Incorporated, Hopkinton, Massachusetts

Contents

chapter 1

Review of Normal Renal Physiology

J. Gary Abuelo

The kidney has three general functions. The **excretory function** is to eliminate the potentially toxic metabolic end products of substances in our diet. Many drugs and their metabolites are also excreted by the kidney. The **homeostatic function** of the kidney is to regulate the body's content of water and ions that make up the internal milieu like sodium (Na^+) and hydrogen (H^+). The **hormonal function** of the kidney is to produce **renin,** which helps regulate blood pressure, total body Na^+ and extracellular volume, to produce **erythropoietin,** which increases red cell production, and to activate **vitamin D,** which maintains calcium levels by stimulating calcium absorption from the gut, the bone, and the renal tubular fluid. In addition, the kidney produces **prosta-glandins** and **kinins,** which are autocoids that act within the kidney itself on renal hemodynamics, Na^+ and water excretion and renin release. This chapter will deal with the kidney's excretory function and its homeostatic role in regulation of water and solutes in the body fluid compartments. Hormonal function will not be covered *per se,* although we briefly discuss renin in this chapter under volume regulation and touch on the role of other hormones in later chapters.

Excretory Function

Waste Excretion

The kidney excretes a majority of the waste products formed from metabolism of the dietary intake. A large number of these products have been identified, but quantitatively the most important ones are 1) **urea** formed from the ammonia given off in protein metabolism, 2) **creatinine** from muscle metabolism, and 3) **uric acid** from purine metabolism. Since there is no way to measure the total blood level of metabolic wastes, serum creatinine level (normal ≤ 1.5 mg/dl) and blood urea nitrogen level (normal ≤ 20 mg/dl) are used to check the efficiency of removal of metabolic wastes. The blood levels of these end products rise slightly if increased dietary intake or increased catabolism of body tissues adds waste products to the body. However, since renal excretion varies with blood levels, this increase in concentration normally results in prompt excretion of the increased load. Impaired renal function leads to accumulation of breakdown products, which may produce deleterious effects on many organ systems, a condition known as **uremia** ("urine in the blood"). This will be discussed in detail in the chapters on **acute and chronic renal failure.**

Waste products generally get into the urine from the blood by filtration in the glomeruli. Due to impermeability of the nephron wall, they tend to remain in the tubular fluid, despite the fact that over 98% of the filtered water and solute is reabsorbed back into the body. Some degradation products, however, such as uric acid, are reabsorbed from the filtrate by the early proximal tubular cells. The cells of the mid-proximal tubule then secrete these products **back into the tubular fluid,** bringing about their elimination in the urine. Tubular secretion is also responsible for urinary excretion of certain waste substances and drugs that are protein bound and thus cannot be filtered by the glomeruli.

Glomerular Filtration

The efficiency of the kidney's excretory function depends on the "processing" of large amounts of blood and the formation of large amounts of filtrate. In fact, the kidneys receive 20% of the cardiac output, more than any other organ, and filter 20% of the plasma flowing through the glomeruli. (The filtration fraction is 0.2.) This high rate of filtration is due to three unique characteristics of the glomerulus. First, the tuft configuration of the glomerular capillaries increases the glomerular **filtering surface** of the two kidneys to 1 M². Second, the pre-glomerular arterioles are relaxed, while the postglomerular arterioles are constricted. This produces higher **hydrostatic pressure** in the glomeruli than in other capillary beds and so maintains a high pressure gradient across the glomerular capillary wall. Third, the glomerular capillary wall has greater **permeability** than other capillaries in the body. Since filtration rate across a capillary bed is the product of surface area, pressure gradient, and permeability, the glomeruli are well-designed to carry out their filtration function. Reduced blood flow may impair glomerular filtration, as will be discussed in the chapter on **renal perfusion disorders.**

The permeability of the glomerular capillary wall is equal for substances with molecular weights of up to 5,000–6,000 daltons and then falls with increasing molecular weight to almost zero at 60,000–70,000 daltons (Fig. 1.1). This means that both metabolic wastes and essential nutrients, such as glucose, amino acids, and vitamins, are filtered freely (i.e. at the same rate as water). Smaller serum proteins (MW <45,000 daltons) are filtered to some degree. Serum albumin (MW 69,000 daltons), IgG (MW 160,000 daltons) and other medium and large serum proteins are filtered only in trace amounts.

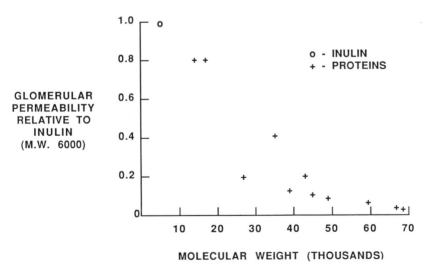

Figure 1.1.   Relation of glomerular permeability of a protein to the molecular weight of that protein. (Adapted with permission from E. Renkin and R. Robinson. Glomerular filtration. N. Engl. J. Med. 1974; 290:785)

Glomerular Filtration Rate

The glomerular filtration rate (GFR) is an important index of renal function in clinical practice. GFR is defined as the rate at which plasma water is filtered across the glomerulus. It is expressed in either ml/min or L/day. When the GFR falls below normal in a patient, he is said to have renal insufficiency or renal failure. The GFR normally depends on the size of an individual and is slightly greater in males. It ranges from 80–120 ml/min in young and middle-aged patients. It tends to fall with advancing age to about one-half of its original value by age 70 years.

The tubule reabsorbs most of the water filtered through the glomerulus, so urine volume may not be used to measure GFR. For estimation of GFR, one needs a substance that is filtered through the glomerulus at the same rate as water and that is quantitatively excreted in the urine, i.e. it is neither reabsorbed nor secreted by the tubular cells. Then the amount of the substance filtered is the same as the amount eliminated in the urine. Also, the amount of the substance filtered is the product of its concentration in the plasma and the amount of plasma water filtered. The amount of water filtered per day (GFR) can be calculated as shown by the following formulas:

For a substance that is neither secreted nor absorbed by the tubule:

$$\text{Substance filtered/day} = \text{Substance excreted in urine/day}$$

$$\text{Plasma level of substance} \times \text{plasma } H_2O \text{ filtered/day}$$
$$= \text{Substance excreted in urine/day;}$$

therefore, GFR or plasma H_2O filtered/day

$$= \frac{\text{Substance excreted in urine/day}}{\text{Plasma level of substance}}$$

Certain exogenous substances such as the polysaccharide **inulin** are ideal to measure GFR and in a research setting can be infused into patients and experimental animals. In clinical practice, the endogenous substance **creatinine,** which is not ideal to measure GFR because of a small amount of tubular secretion, is commonly used to estimate GFR, because it does not have to be infused:

$$\text{GFR} \sim \frac{\text{Creatinine excreted/day}}{\text{Plasma creatinine level}}$$

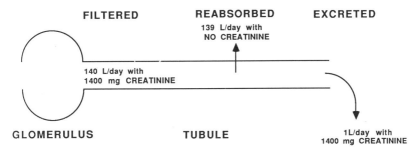

FILTERED   REABSORBED   EXCRETED

139 L/day with
NO CREATININE

140 L/day with
1400 mg CREATININE

GLOMERULUS   TUBULE   1L/day with
1400 mg CREATININE

Figure 1.2. Diagram showing the fate of the water and creatinine that is filtered by the glomeruli each day.

For example, if a 24-hour urine collection contains 1,400 mg of creatinine and the concentration in the plasma is 1 mg/dl (same as 10 mg/L), then the glomerular filtration rate would be 1,400 mg/day ÷ 10 mg/L or 140 L/day[a]. This 140 L/day is the **creatinine clearance (Ccr),** i.e. the rate of removal of creatinine from the blood in terms of the amount of blood totally cleared per day or per unit time. In fact, almost all of the 140 L is reabsorbed by the tubule without creatinine back into the body (Fig. 1.2). Due to tubular secretion, Ccr is slightly more (~10% more) than true GFR as determined by inulin clearance.

A practical consideration in determining Ccr is to verify that the urine collection is complete. This can be checked by looking at the total creatinine in the specimen, which is equal to daily creatinine production and under steady state conditions is constant in any patient from day to day. This amount should be about 1–1.5 gm/day in most adults of average size.

After determining Ccr, one must consider the size and age of the patient. The normal values of 80–120 cc/min would be too low for a large man and too high for children and many elderly patients. Ccr can be corrected for body surface area in children and large individuals by normalizing to 1.73 M^2, according to this formula: corrected Ccr = measured Ccr × 1.73 M^2 ÷ body surface area. Body surface is estimated from height and weight using a table or nomogram.

---

[a]N.B. The laboratory reports plasma creatinine concentration in mg/dl. This must be multiplied by 10 to convert it to mg/L before using it in the formula for Ccr. The Ccr expressed by L/day may simply be converted to ml/min by dividing by 1.44, i.e. Ccr (L/day) [1000 ml/L ÷ (24 hours/day × 60 min/hour)].

Plasma Creatinine Level

Assume a person has two equally functioning kidneys, a Ccr (GFR) of 140 L/day, and a plasma creatinine (Pcr) of 10 mg/L (same as 1 mg/dl). If he were to donate a kidney to a relative with renal failure, his Ccr would immediately fall by one-half to 70 L/day. The rate of creatinine excretion per day (Ccr × Pcr) would also fall by one-half from 1400 to 700 mg/day. Since creatinine continues to be produced from muscle at a constant rate, creatinine will begin to accumulate in the body, and Pcr will rise. When Pcr reaches twice its original value, creatinine excretion (½ original Ccr × 2 × original Pcr) will again equal the production rate, and the Pcr will remain at this new higher steady state value (Fig. 1.3).

Similarly, any reduction in Ccr will be followed by a rise in Pcr to a new steady state level at which urine excretion of creatinine again equals creatinine production, which is constant in any individual. This relationship is shown when our formula for Ccr is rewritten to indicate that Ccr is proportional to 1/steady state Pcr:

$$Ccr = \frac{Creatinine\ excrete/day}{Pcr}$$

$$Ccr = Constant \times \frac{1}{Pcr}$$

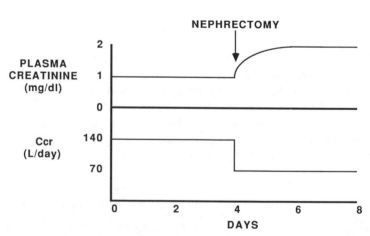

Figure 1.3. Graph showing new steady state plasma creatinine concentration after loss of GFR caused by a nephrectomy.

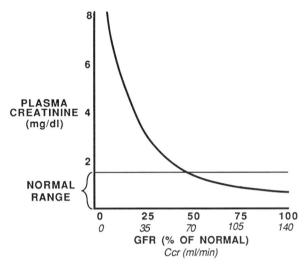

Figure 1.4. Relation between GFR and steady state Pcr in a hypothetical individual with progressive renal disease.

This mathematical relationship is a hyperbola. When Ccr falls below normal in diseased kidneys, the rise in Pcr is initially small. In fact, the GFR could fall by one-half and the Pcr may not rise out of the normal range (≤ 1.5 mg/dl). For example, if the Ccr fell from 140 to 70 L/day, the Pcr might double from 0.7 to 1.4 mg/dl. Subsequent falls in Ccr beyond this point would be accompanied by a more substantial rise in Pcr (Fig. 1.4).

The rise of steady state Pcr with falls in GFR has led to the clinical practice of estimating renal function from Pcr alone without bothering to collect a timed urine sample. A Pcr well within the normal range (≤ 1.2 mg/dl) is taken to indicate normal GFR. Values of 1.3–1.6 mg/dl could either reflect borderline renal function or increased creatinine production in a muscular individual. Higher Pcr (≥ 1.7 mg/dl) indicates renal failure. Also changes in Pcr appear to reliably signal an improvement or deterioration in GFR.

If one could estimate creatinine production rate from the size, age and sex of an individual, i.e. without collection of a 24-hour urine, then one could use Pcr to determine Ccr from the equation: Ccr = creatinine excretion per day/Pcr, which equals creatinine production per day/Pcr. Many such formulas for estimation of creatinine clearance have been proposed. The most widely used is that of Cockcroft and Gault:

Creatinine production/day (mg/day)

$$= \frac{(140 - \text{age}) \times \text{body wt(kg)} \times 0.85^*}{5}$$

Creatinine clearance (ml/min)

$$= \frac{(140 - \text{age}) \times \text{body wt(kg)} \times 0.85^*}{72 \times \text{Pcr (mg/dl)}}$$

*if patient is a female

Can you derive the second formula?

Blood Urea Nitrogen Level

The serum level of another metabolic waste product, **urea,** has been used to estimate renal function in the same way as has the level of serum creatinine (Scr[b]). This level is expressed as blood urea nitrogen concentration (BUN), and normal values are ≤ 20 mg/dl. The increase of BUN and Scr in the blood is called **azotemia** ("nitrogen in the blood").

Considerable reabsorption of filtered urea across the tubular wall leaves only about 50% in the urine, i.e. clearance of urea (Curea) is only 50% of GFR. As long as the percent of reabsorption is constant, changes in Curea parallel those of Ccr. Similarly, when GFR falls, BUN usually rises proportionately to Scr, maintaining a BUN/Scr ratio of 10:1 to 15:1 under usual circumstances. However, when azotemia is associated with slow tubular flow rates, the longer contact between the filtrate and tubular wall enhances reabsorption of urea and raises the BUN/Scr ratio to 20:1 or higher. This is typical of renal failure caused by volume depletion or urinary outflow obstruction and, in fact, should make one consider these diagnoses. Unfortunately, increased urea production can also increase BUN/Scr ratios. This may be seen when high protein loads are absorbed from the gut, such as with gastrointestinal bleeding or high-protein meals, or when protein is broken down or not synthesized due to administration of corticosteroids or tetracyclines.

---

[b]Clinical laboratories usually measure extracellular creatinine concentrations in samples of serum (Scr) rather than plasma (Pcr). Scr equals Pcr, and the two terms can be used interchangeably.

"Conservatory Function"

The kidney is able to clear metabolic wastes from the blood efficiently, while conserving cells, protein, and nutrients. Cells and proteins with molecular weights >70,000 daltons do not cross the glomerular capillary wall. Smaller proteins, peptides, amino acids, and glucose are, however, filtered to a variable degree. The proximal tubule actively reabsorbs these valuable substances, minimizing their loss in the urine.

Glomerular damage may permit red blood cells and large quantities of protein to enter the filtrate and appear in the urine (**hematuria** and **proteinuria**) and may impair GFR. This will be discussed in the chapter on **glomerular disorders.** Rarely, tubular disorders lead to urinary loss of small proteins, amino acids and glucose. Beyond the mention of renal tubular acidosis in the chapter on **acid-base disorders** and cystinuria in the chapter on **disorders of urinary outflow,** these conditions will not be covered.

Body Fluid Compartments

Volume of Compartments (Fig. 1.5)

Total volume of body fluids **(total body water)** is about 60% of total body weight, being lower in individuals with a high percentage of adipose tissue, which contains very little water. Approximately two-thirds of this total body water is inside cells **(intracellular water);** one-third outside cells **(extracellular water).** The latter compartment is subdivided into **intravascular fluid (plasma),** which is about one-fourth of the extracellular fluid, and **interstitial fluid,** which makes up the remaining three-fourths. About 2% of total body water is **transcellular water.** This is fluid contained in separate places such as cerebrospinal fluid, synovial fluid, intraocular fluid, and fluid contained in the gastrointestinal tract.

Water and solutes pass with varying ease from one body fluid compartment to another in continuous dynamic equilibrium. The Starling forces, which vary in magnitude from tissue to tissue in the body, continually drive fluid out of the capillaries. On average, there is a net oncotic pressure due to plasma proteins directed inwards of 20.7 mm Hg and a net hydrostatic pressure directed outwards of 21 mm Hg. The resulting outward force of 0.3 mm Hg moves fluid from the plasma into the interstitial space. The size of this space, however, is relatively

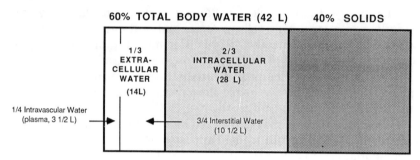

Figure 1.5.   Body fluid compartments in an average 70-kg man.

constant since fluid is drained back to the veins by the lymphatics at the same rate. The distribution of the extracellular fluid between the intravascular space and the interstitium depends on this balance between fluid filtration from the capillaries and lymphatic return to the veins.

Tonicity and Solute Content of Body Compartments

The body maintains a constant osmolarity by mechanisms that will be discussed later on in this chapter. Most cellular membranes are freely permeable to water. When the osmolarity of one compartment is altered, water shifts rapidly to equalize osmolarity differences. Consequently, all body fluid compartments have the same osmolarity. The fluid volume of the various compartments is a reflection, then, of the amount of osmotic particles in that compartment and is not dependent on some ability of the cells selectively to hold water in one or another of these compartments. One exception to this is the nephron, certain parts of which are impermeable to water.

The term **tonicity,** or the effective osmotic pressure equivalent of a solution, is often used interchangeably with **osmolarity,** since the osmolarity of body fluids is usually about the same as the tonicity. This is because most solutes in the body, such as glucose, sodium (Na^+), potassium (K^+), and chloride (Cl^-), produce osmotic pressure differences due to their inability to freely move across membranes. However, this is not the case with a solute like urea. Since it can freely cross a membrane, it will achieve equal concentrations on both sides of the membrane and will not exert any effective osmotic pressure at all. The tonicity of a urea solution will be zero! Therefore, solutions with high urea content, as in the medulla of the kidney, have less tonicity than osmolarity.

The net osmotic effect of the intra- and extracellular solutes is an **osmolarity** of about 285 mOsm/L. Clinically, the osmotic pressure of plasma and urine is usually measured with an osmometer, which works by determining the depression of freezing point by the solutes in solution. The results are reported in mOsm/kg, also known as **osmolality**. Because of low solute concentrations in the body fluids, the difference between osmolarity and osmolality is negligible, and the terms are used interchangeably.

As can be seen in Table 1.1, the most important extracellular osmotic particles are the electrolytes, Na^+, Cl^-, and bicarbonate (HCO_3^-), while the most important intracellular osmotic particles are K^+ and phosphate.

The partition of ions between the cells and the extracellular space depends on their continuous active and passive transport across cell membranes. The Na^+ - K^+ pump, which maintains low Na^+ and high K^+ concentrations in the cells, is the most important of many transport systems. The distribution of nonionic osmotic particles, such as glucose and amino acids, depends on both membrane transport and

Table 1.1.
Principal Ions in the Body Fluid Compartments[a]

	Cations (mEq/L)					Anions (mEq/L)			
	Na^+	K^+	Ca^{2+}	Mg^{2+}	H^{+b}	Cl^-	HCO_3^-	PO_4	Protein
Plasma	142	4.3	2.5	1.1	0.000040	104	24	2.0	14.0[c]
Interstitial fluid	145	4.4	2.4	1.1	0.000040	117	27	2.3	0
Intracellular fluid (variable)	12	150	4.0	34	0.000080	4.0	12	40.0	54.0[c]

[a]Modified from B.D. Rose. Clinical physiology of acid-base and electrolyte disorders, 2nd ed. New York: McGraw-Hill Book Company, 1984:23.
[b]H^+ concentration is included in table and expressed in mEq/L to emphasize that it is orders of magnitude less than that of other ions and that osmotic effect is negligible.
[c]Osmotic effect of protein is negligible, despite the large number of anions, since protein has relatively few molecules (osmotic particles), each with many anionic groups such as $-COO^-$.

metabolism. The volume of cells and, consequently, of the whole intra-cellular space reflects the number of osmotic particles maintained within the cells by multiple metabolic and transport processes. Some cells, such as those in the brain, may regulate their volume by altera-tion of intracellular osmotic particles, but little is known about such processes elsewhere in the body.

H^+ Concentration of Body Compartments

Normal extracellular pH is 7.40, which corresponds to a hydrogen ion (H^+) concentration of 40 nEq/L. Intracellular pH is somewhat lower than extracellular pH and varies from organ to organ. It changes in tandem with extracellular pH.

The relation of H^+ concentration to pH is given by the following formulas:

$$
\begin{aligned}
\text{By definition,} \quad -\log H^+ &= pH \\
\log H^+ &= -pH \\
H^+ &= \text{anti log} \, (-pH) \\
\text{for pH} = 7.40, \, H^+ &= \text{anti log} \, (-7.40) \\
&= \text{anti log} \, (0.60 - 8) \\
&= 4 \times 10^{-8} \, \text{Eq/L} \\
&\quad (\times 10^9 \, \text{nEq/Eq}) \\
&= 40 \, \text{nEq/L}
\end{aligned}
$$

The relation between H^+ concentration and pH approximates a straight line in and near the physiologic range (Fig. 1.6). Table 1.2 shows how H^+ concentration can be estimated from pH, assuming a 1 nEq/L change in H^+ for each 0.01 change in pH.

Potassium Content of Body Compartments

Potassium (K^+) is the major intracellular cation. Because of the extremely low extracellular K^+ concentration ($\sim$4 mEq/L) compared to the intracellular concentration (as high as 150 mEq/L) and because intracellular volume is twice extracellular volume, only about 2% of total body K^+ is in the extracellular space. The wide difference in K^+ concentrations between the two spaces is the result of the membrane enzyme, Na^+ - K^+ ATPase, which transports K^+ into cells and removes Na^+. Sodium constantly leaks into and K^+ out of the cell down their respective concentration gradients, which necessitates the constant activity of this pump.

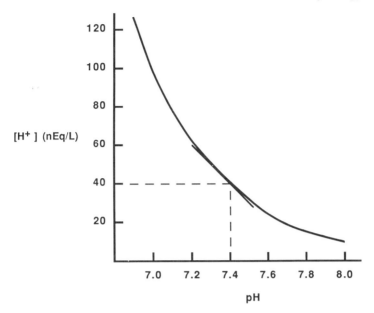

Figure 1.6. The relation between H^+ concentration and pH. Both the true curve and a straight line approximation (ΔH^+ concentration nEq/L = 100ΔpH) between pH 7.2 and 7.5 are shown. (Modified from Cohen JJ, Kassirer JP, Gennari FJ, et al., Acid-Base. Boston: Little Brown & Company, 1982:410.)

Table 1.2.
Comparison of True and Estimated
Hydrogen Ion Concentrations

pH	True H^+ (nEq/L)	Estimated H^+ (nEq/L)
7.20	63	60
7.30	50	50
7.40	40	40
7.50	32	30
7.60	25	20

Renal Regulation of Body Fluid Compartments

Extracellular Volume (Sodium) Regulation

The kidney regulates the body's extracellular volume through its handling of Na^+, the salts of which constitute the vast majority of solutes in this space. When Na^+ is added to the body, as by eating potato chips, it goes into the extracellular volume and transiently raises tonicity. Since the body maintains constant tonicity by regulating body water content, water will be accumulated via the thirst mechanism and renal conservation of water. As tonicity returns to normal, extracellular volume will increase slightly. On the other hand, when Na^+ is lost from the body[c], water will be excreted by the kidneys to normalize tonicity, and extracellular volume will fall. These increases and decreases in extracellular volume are reflected in parallel changes in intravascular volume and, ultimately, in cardiac output and perfusion of the organs of the body. Normally, extracellular volume is about 20% of body weight, but this is not usually measured in the clinical setting. When extracellular volume falls below normal, the ensuing decrease in blood pressure and organ perfusion may cause shock. Conversely, when extracellular volume rises above normal, hypertension (see chapter on **hypertension**) and circulatory congestion may occur. Thus, the regulation of Na^+ homeostasis by the kidney is one of its most critical functions.

Volume Receptors

The body senses loss of intravascular volume through receptors in the cardiopulmonary circulation and carotid sinus, resulting in **sympathetic neural signals** to the kidney. Baroreceptors in the afferent glomerular arteriole also sense reduction in perfusion pressure. This leads to release of **renin,** a proteolytic enzyme, from the juxtaglomerular cells. Increased sympathetic neural tone to the kidney and decreased NaCl delivery to the macular densa of the distal convoluted tubule as a result of reduced GFR also stimulate renin release. Renin cleaves a decapeptide, **angiotensin I,** from a circulating renin substrate, **angiotensinogen,** which is produced by the liver (Fig. 1.7). A converting enzyme, found in the plasma, lung, kidney and other tissues, converts

---

[c]Sodium is never lost from the body without water. However, if one loses a liter of diarrhea with 50 mEq/L of sodium and ingests a liter of water, the net effect is pure sodium loss.

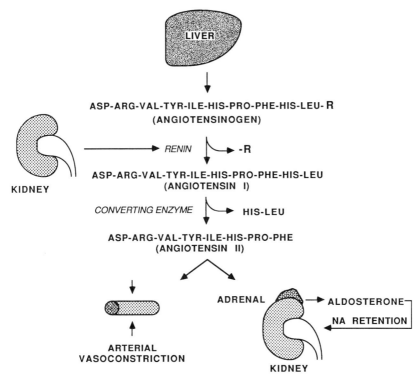

Figure 1.7. Renal-angiotensin-aldosterone system. (Modified from Ballermann BJ, Levenson DJ, Brenner BM. (Chapter 9) Renin, angiotensin, kinins, prostaglandins, and leukotrienes. In: Brenner BM and Rector FC, Jr. eds. The kidney. 3rd ed. Philadelphia: W. B. Saunders Company, 1986:282.)

angiotensin I to an octapeptide, **angiotensin II,** which raises blood pressure by arterial vasoconstriction. It also stimulates the release from the adrenal cortex of **aldosterone,** a steroid hormone that stimulates renal Na^+ retention. In addition, **atrial natriuretic factor** may be released from the cardiac atria in response to volume expansion. This hormone increases Na^+ excretion by raising GFR and by reducing tubular reabsorption of Na^+. It also opposes renin and aldosterone secretion and the Na^+-retaining action of aldosterone.

Normal Sodium Balance

Normally, dietary Na^+, about 150 mEq/day, is excreted in the urine. With changes in Na^+ intake, minimum alterations in circulating volume are sensed and urine Na⁺ excretion rises or falls to maintain extracellular volume. The homeostatic range is so great that the kidney can match dietary Na⁺ intake ranging from <1 to over 1,000 mEq/day by appropriate changes in urine Na⁺ output.

Renal Sodium Handling

Renal Na⁺ excretion begins with the filtration of about 140 L each day containing 19,600 mEq Na⁺ (140 L/day × 140 mEq/L). The tubules then reabsorb almost all of this filtered Na⁺ (usually 99% or more), leaving about 150 mEq to be excreted under normal circumstances. Seventy percent of filtered Na⁺ is reabsorbed in the proximal tubule. In order to preserve electroneutrality, it must be reabsorbed with Cl⁻ or "in exchange for" H⁺. Twenty percent of filtered Na⁺ is reabsorbed in the thick ascending limb of the loop of Henle and in the distal convoluted tubule along with Cl⁻, and 9% in the collecting duct either along with Cl⁻ or "in exchange for" K⁺ or H⁺ (Fig. 1.8).

The mechanisms controlling the urine excretion rate of Na⁺ are only partly understood, but appear to take at least three forms (Fig. 1.9). Following a fall in Na⁺ intake, ongoing urine Na⁺ excretion leads to a slight fall in extracellular volume, cardiac output and blood pressure,

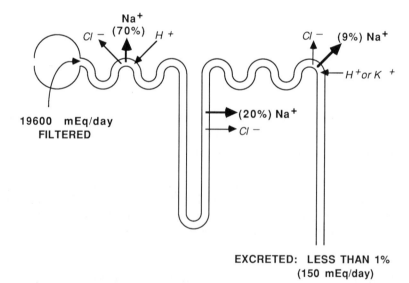

Figure 1.8.   Overview of filtration and reabsorption of Na⁺ by the kidney.

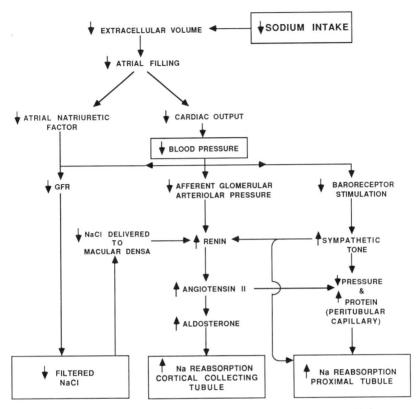

Figure 1.9.   The mechanisms involved in the reduction of urine Na^+ excretion in response to reduced Na^+ intake.

which reduce GFR and, consequently, the filtered Na^+ load. The GFR may also be reduced in response to low atrial natriuretic factor levels, which fall as circulating volume decreases. Second, increased aldosterone stimulates reabsorption of Na^+ in the cortical collecting duct in exchange for K^+ and H^+. Third, proximal tubular Na^+ reabsorption increases in response to reduced circulating volume by a mechanism called the third factor. Actually more than one process is involved. Increased sympathetic tone may be one such mechanism, as may reduced hydrostatic pressure and increased protein content in peritubular capillaries. These changes in capillary hydraulic and oncotic forces increase fluid uptake by the capillaries and secondarily enhance proximal tubule Na^+ and water reabsorption. Conversely, in the face of increased Na^+ intake, the reversal of these mechanisms would favor high glomerular filtration of Na^+ and low tubular reabsorption.

The continuous action of Na^+ regulation by the kidney in response to volume receptors and neural and hormonal signals maintains extracellular volume and, in turn, circulating volume. In certain disease states, the circulating or intravascular volume may be abnormally expanded, which is called **volume overload,** or abnormally reduced, which is called **volume depletion.** These disturbances in volume will be considered in the next chapter on **volume disorders.**

Body Tonicity (Water) Regulation

When water is added to the body, as when a person drinks a glass of water, osmolarity falls first in the extracellular space, and then, as cells take up the water, in the intracellular space (Fig. 1.10). Conversely, when water is lost from the body, as occurs through skin and urine losses when one has limited access to water, osmolarity increases in the extracellular space and, then, as cells give up water, in the intracellular space. The kidney counteracts these changes through greater or lesser excretion of ingested water and the body's osmolarity normally varies little despite wide ranges of water intake. However, if extracellular osmolarity should fall below normal (280–290 mOsm/L), the body's cells may swell significantly. If extracellular osmolarity rises above normal, cells shrink. In the central nervous system, marked changes of cell volume can cause mental changes, seizures, and death. Thus, the kidney's role in maintenance of body osmolarity within normal limits through regulation of water excretion is an essential one.

Tonicity Receptors

Receptors for plasma tonicity are in the hypothalamus. They react to hypertonicity by stimulating thirst and by releasing **antidiuretic hormone (ADH, arginine vasopressin)** from the posterior pituitary gland. Thirst and ADH release are also stimulated by certain nonosmotic factors, such as moderately severe volume depletion. ADH is an octapeptide synthesized in the hypothalamus and transported to the pituitary gland for storage and secretion. It reduces water excretion by the kidney.

Normal Water Balance

Normally, each day we lose 100 ml of water in the stool and evaporate 900 ml from the skin and respiratory tract. These **insensible**

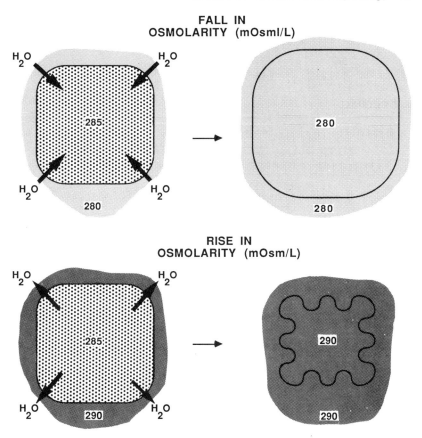

Figure 1.10. Depiction of cell volume changes that occur in response to changes in extracellular osmolarity.

losses are partly balanced by 400 ml of water produced from the oxidation of carbohydrate, fat and protein, leaving an extrarenal net loss of 600 ml/day. In addition, there is an obligatory urine output of 500 ml/day. Consequently, we must take in a minimum of 1,100 ml/day to prevent dehydration. Normally we drink about 1,500 ml/day (this is very variable) and ingest another 800 ml/day in water contained in food (some vegetables are almost 100% water). As a result, the kidney excretes 1,700 ml/day to maintain water balance in a typical individual (Fig. 1.11).

A reduction in water intake with continued urinary water excretion will lead to a rise in plasma osmolarity. Through the action of ADH,

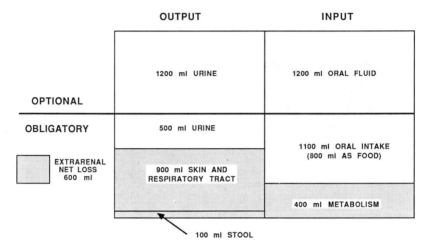

urine water output will fall in order to maintain plasma osmolarity. In addition, the increased osmolarity will lead to stimulation of thirst. In contrast, increased water intake will lead to opposite changes. The range of the kidney's water output to accommodate the variations in intake may range from 500 cc to well over 12 L.

Along with the water excreted, the kidney must eliminate about 600 mOsm/day of urinary solute principally in the form of urea and salts of Na^+ and K^+. In fact, it is the kidney's limits of dilution (50 mOsm/L) and concentration (1200 mOsm/L) combined with this osmotic load that determines the range of possible daily urine outputs: 0.5L (600 mOsm ÷ 1200 mOsm/L) to 12L (600 mOsm ÷ 50 mOsm/L). Obligatory urine output is 500 cc/day, since this is the minimum volume of urine needed to excrete the body's daily urinary solute at maximum concentration.

Renal Water Handling

The kidney achieves this range of urinary concentrations and volumes by first producing a large amount of dilute fluid in the loop of Henle and distal convoluted tubule (Fig. 1.12). When this passes through the highly concentrated medulla in the presence of maximum ADH, most of the water will be reabsorbed, leaving only a small volume of highly concentrated urine to be excreted. In contrast, in the absence of ADH, only about one-half of the water is reabsorbed, and

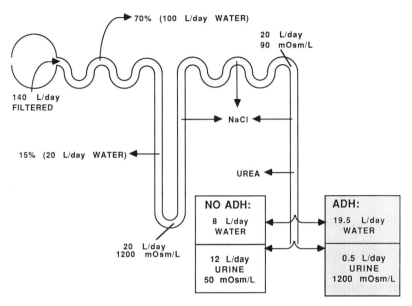

Figure 1.12. Overview of water handling by the kidney under absent or maximum physiologic ADH levels.

the tubular fluid remains dilute due to the active NaCl reabsorption that is also taking place in the collecting duct. Under normal conditions, urine volumes are regulated by ADH levels in the intermediate range.

The medullary concentration is high (1400 mOsm/L) partly because the ascending limb of the loop of Henle actively reabsorbs NaCl without water into the medullary interstitium (Fig. 1.12). Medullary concentration is also high because large amounts of urea enter the inner medulla from the collecting tubule. Urea becomes very concentrated in this part of the collecting tubule, because the tubular fluid has come from the cortical and outer medullary collecting tubule, which are impermeable to urea but are sites of substantial passive water reabsorption under the influence of ADH. In the inner medulla, the collecting tubule become permeable to urea, which passively moves out of the duct down its concentration gradient. The high concentrations of NaCl and urea are not washed out of the medulla because medullary blood flow is low and the capillaries of the vasa recta are arranged in a hairpin or countercurrent exchange configuration.

Of the 140 L/day of fluid filtered at the glomerulus, it is thought that about 70% or 100 L/day are reabsorbed isosmotically in the proximal tubule due to the osmotic gradient formed by active Na^+ reabsorption. Another 20 L/day are reabsorbed passively into the more concentrated medulla in the descending loop of Henle, which is permeable to water and relatively impermeable to solutes. In this process 20 L/day of highly concentrated tubular fluid reach the papillary tip (hairpin turn) of the loop of Henle. As it ascends, the loop of Henle becomes impermeable to water. Salt is reabsorbed passively in the inner medulla (driven by very high Na^+ concentrations) and then actively in the thick ascending limb of the outer medulla and cortex. In the process the tubular fluid becomes hypotonic to plasma. Salt reabsorption without water continues in the distal convoluted tubule such that the collecting duct receives 20 L/day of dilute tubular fluid with concentrations below 100 mOsm/L. Now, depending on the concentration of ADH present, tubular permeability to water increases, allowing passive reabsorption of water first in the isotonic cortex and then in the hypertonic medulla. This water reabsorption varies in amount from 8 to 19½L with increasing ADH levels, leading to urine volumes varying from 12L/day or more down to 0.5L/day (Fig. 1.12). Due to reabsorption of Na^+ and urea by the collecting duct, final urine concentration may be as low as 50 mOsm/L in the absence of ADH. With maximum physiologic levels of ADH urine concentration approaches that of the medullary interstitium.

The continuous regulation of body water content and tonicity by the kidney in response to hypothalamic signals via ADH maintains constant body tonicity and, in turn, intracellular volume. In disease states, body water may be abnormally depleted, leading to **hypertonic dehydration** or may be excessive, leading to **hyponatremia.** These disturbances will be considered in the chapter on **tonicity disorders.**

Acid-Base Regulation

Most nonvegetarian diets are metabolized to a variety of acids. For example, sulfur-containing amino acids yield sulfuric acid and phosphorus-containing substances yield phosphoric acid. Acid added to the body after a nonvegetarian meal or from other sources lowers pH in the intra- and extracellular spaces. In contrast, vegetarian diets generally are metabolized to a variety of bases. For example, Na citrate yields $NaHCO_3$, which is the metabolic equivalent of NaOH. Alkali added to the body after such a meal or from other sources raises pH in the intra- and extracellular spaces.

The kidney maintains a constant body pH in the face of these dietary loads through the excretion of various amounts of either acid or alkali. Processes that raise the pH of the body (called **alkalosis**) or decrease the pH of the body (called **acidosis**) may interfere with the function of cells and enzymes and may have deleterious effects on the heart, brain and other organ systems. Therefore, the preservation of normal body pH (7.37–7.42) and H^+ concentration (38–43 nEq/L) is one of the kidney's most important functions.

Buffers

When either acid or alkali is added to the body, their disequilibrating effect on pH is greatly reduced by proteins and certain weak acids and their salts. These act as **buffers** by taking up H^+ when acid is added or releasing H^+ when alkali is added. The most important buffer in the body is the **carbonic acid/bicarbonate (H_2CO_3/HCO_3^-) buffer system.** With the addition of acid, HCO_3^- is consumed and turned to CO_2 and water. With the addition of alkali to the body, CO_2 and water are converted to H_2CO_3, which neutralizes the alkali and is converted to HCO_3^-. Buffers will be discussed further in the chapter on **acid-base disorders.**

$$HCO_3^-/\ H_2CO_3 \quad \textbf{BUFFER SYSTEM}$$

ADDITION OF ACID: HCl   NaCl

$$NaHCO_3 \rightleftarrows H_2CO_3 \rightleftarrows CO_2 + H_2O$$

ADDITION OF BASE: H_2O NaOH

pH Receptors

There are pH receptors in the brain that control ventilation, but there are no known pH receptors in the body that affect renal acid excretion. The kidney changes its excretion of acid or base mainly according to extracellular pH.

Normal Acid-Base Balance

Normally, the kidney excretes the 70–100 mEq acid produced each day from metabolic conversion of dietary precursors. With addition of more or less H^+ to the body, acid excretion rises or falls to maintain body pH constant. If, as in vegetarians, greater or lesser amounts of alkali are produced, acid is not excreted, but instead varying amounts of alkali appear in the urine. In fact, up to 700 mEq/day of either acid or base may be excreted in the urine in order to maintain acid-base homeostasis.

Renal Acid-Base Handling

It should be noted that little acid or base per se is excreted. To do so would require the elaboration of urine with pH's ranging from 1 to 12. The kidney is incapable of producing urine at these extreme pH's. Instead, the urine contains the metabolic equivalent of H^+ or hydroxide (OH^-) ions. For example, instead of H^+, NH_4^+ and $H_2PO_4^-$ are produced and excreted by the kidney. Instead of OH^-, HCO_3^- is produced in the body and excreted by the kidney.

EXCRETION OF ACID

(IN KIDNEY) $HCL + NH_3 \longrightarrow NH_4CL$

(IN KIDNEY) $HCL + Na_2HPO_4 \longrightarrow NaCl + NaH_2PO_4$

EXCRETION OF ALKALI

(IN EXTRACELLULAR SPACE) $NaOH + H_2CO_3 \longrightarrow NaHCO_3 + H_2O$

$$H_2O + CO_2 \rightleftarrows$$

The kidney achieves its range of acid or base excretion by first producing a glomerular filtrate with a large amount of base equivalent ($NaHCO_3$), which is then reabsorbed (through the secretion of H^+) by the tubular cells. If an alkaline urine is to be produced, the reabsorption is incomplete, allowing $NaHCO_3$ to be excreted in the urine. If an acid urine is to be produced, enough H^+ is secreted not only to completely reabsorb $NaHCO_3$, but also to yield an acidic urine.

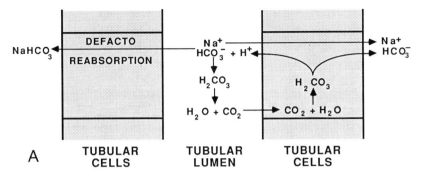

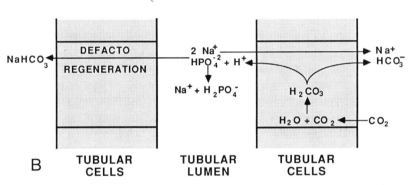

Figure 1.13. (A) Tubular **reabsorption** of $NaHCO_3$. The secretion of H^+ into the tubular lumen converts HCO_3^- to CO_2 which diffuses into the tubular cell and is reconverted to HCO_3^-. The HCO_3^- diffuses into the peritubular interstitium and then to the blood along with Na^+ reabsorbed from the tubular lumen. (B) Tubular **regeneration** of HCO_3^-. The secretion of H^+ into the tubular lumen converts HPO_4^{-2} to $H_2PO_4^-$ and does not produce CO_2. The tubular cell takes CO_2 from the interstitium and uses it to generate new HCO_3^-. This HCO_3^- diffuses into the interstitium along with Na^+ reaborbed from the tubular lumen.

Each day the glomerular filtrate ordinarily contains about 3,360 mEq $NaHCO_3$ (140 L $\times$ 24 mEq/L). The proximal and distal tubular cells reabsorb this in effect by reabsorbing Na^+ and simultaneously secreting H^+ into the tubular lumen (Fig. 1.13A). The secreted H^+ brings about the reabsorption of HCO_3^- by a circuitous route. First, the H^+ "destroys" intraluminal (filtered) HCO_3^- by combining with it and converting it to H_2CO_3, which then dissociates to water and carbon dioxide (CO_2). Next, the CO_2 diffuses into the tubular cell, where it recombines with water, is converted to HCO_3^-, and passes into the peritubular interstitium. The reabsorbed $NaHCO_3$ then diffuses into the blood.

The proximal tubule cell is incapable of secreting H^+ against a large gradient. Nevertheless, the proximal tubule secretes large quantities of H^+ (and reabsorbs large quantities of HCO_3^-) because the enzyme, carbonic anhydrase, at the luminal surface of the cells facilitates conversion of H_2CO_3 to water and CO_2, preventing marked accumulation of H^+. By the end of the proximal tubule, 80–90% of $NaHCO_3$ has been reabsorbed, but pH has fallen only to 6.8. The distal convoluted and collecting tubules continue the reabsorption of $NaHCO_3$. This will be incomplete after an alkaline load, since high pH reduces H^+ secretion by the tubular cells. The urine will have pH greater than 7 and sufficient $NaHCO_3$ to reduce body pH to normal.

If an acid load has been added to the body, then the decreased extracellular pH stimulates H^+ secretion, driving final urine pH as low as 4.5 in the process. At a tubular fluid pH of 6.0 reclamation of $NaHCO_3$ is virtually complete, but H^+ secretion continues. As urine pH falls along the nephron, tubular fluid Na_2HPO_4, rather than $NaHCO_3$, begins to take up H^+ in the proximal tubule and may buffer up to 40 mEq/day in a maximally acid urine (pH 4.5–5.0). Also cells of the proximal convoluted tubules produce NH_3, which diffuses throughout the kidney and combines with H^+ in the tubular fluid. Normally about 40 mEq H^+ combines with 40 mmol NH_3/day. Both NH_3 production and H^+ secretion rise with increasing acid loads, so that up to 250 mEq H^+/day may be excreted as NH_4^+. This acid excretion in the form of $H_2PO_4^-$ and NH_4^+ matches the ingested acid load and thereby restores acid base homeostasis. Figure 1.14 depicts how urine HCO_3^- and acid excretion vary at different urine pH in a typical individual.

The distal nephron also restores acid-base homeostasis by generating new HCO_3^- to replace the HCO_3^- that was consumed when the acid load was first buffered in the body. This new HCO_3^- is created when secreted H^+ reacts with HPO_4^{-2} and NH_3 rather than converting intraluminal HCO_3^- to CO_2. Consequently, the distal tubule must generate HCO_3^- from the body's CO_2 as opposed to from CO_2 derived from luminal HCO_3^- (Fig. 1.13B).

The continued maintenance of body pH (H^+ concentration) by the kidney is essential for the proper function of enzymes and cells. In disease states, alkalosis or acidosis may cause body pH to rise or fall out

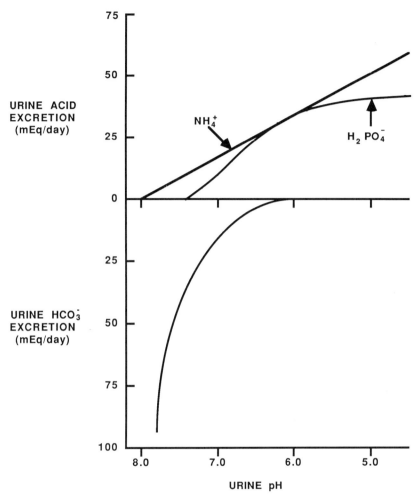

Figure 1.14. Representative urine excretions of HCO_3^- and acid (as $H_2PO_2^-$ and NH_4^+) at varying urine pH.

of the normal range. These pH disturbances will be considered in the chapter on **acid-base disorders.**

Potassium Regulation

Dietary K^+ is readily absorbed from the small intestine and transiently raises plasma (extracellular) K^+ levels. On the other hand, during fasting, normal losses of K^+ in the stool and urine tend to lower plasma levels. These changes in extracellular K^+ concentration stimulate the body's cells to take up or release K^+, so as to prevent a dangerous elevation or fall of plasma levels. In addition, the kidney increases or decreases urine K^+ excretion greatly in response to these changes, thereby maintaining normal body K^+ content and plasma concentration (normally 3.5 to 5 mEq/L). If abnormalities of K^+ homeostasis lead to depletion or overload of body K^+ and attendant changes in plasma concentration (**hypokalemia or hyperkalemia**), deleterious effects on muscle strength and cardiac rhythm may be seen.

Potassium Receptors

There is no receptor for K^+ levels per se. However, the zona granulosa cells of the adrenal gland raise aldosterone secretion in response to a small rise in plasma K^+ level, and vice versa. At the kidney, aldosterone promotes K^+ secretion into the tubular lumen and, thus, plays a major role in K^+ homeostasis.

Potassium Balance

Normally, 60–120 mEq K^+ are absorbed from the diet and excreted by the kidney daily. The range of urinary K^+ excreted in order to regulate body K^+ may vary from 10 to 15 mEq to several hundred mEq/ day.

Renal Potassium Handling

Renal excretion of K^+ paradoxically does not depend on glomerular filtration, since filtered K^+ is essentially all reabsorbed in the proximal tubule and loop of Henle. Urine K^+ excretion is, instead, dependent on K^+ secretion into the lumen by the cells of the distal convoluted tubule, the medullary and, especially, the cortical collecting duct. This latter segment responds to elevated plasma K^+ and aldosterone levels by increasing K^+ secretion. In certain disease states, the serum K^+ concentration[d] rises above or falls below the normal range (3.5–5 mEq/L). These disturbances will be considered in the chapter on **potassium disorders**.

---

[d]The serum K^+ concentration is equal or slightly higher than the plasma K^+ concentration. They are assumed to be equal and representative of extracellular K^+ concentration for most clinical purposes and K^+ concentration is usually measured in specimens of serum rather than plasma.

Suggested Readings

Alpern RJ. Regulation and disorders of extracellular fluid volume. In: Brenner B, Coe FL, Rector FC, Jr, eds. Renal physiology in health and disease. Philadelphia: W.B. Saunders Company, 1987:84–111.

Berry CA. Transport functions of the renal tubules. In: Brenner B, Coe FL, Rector FC, Jr, eds. Renal physiology in health and disease. Philadelphia: W.B. Saunders Company, 1987:27–56.

Cogan MG. Acid-base homeostasis. In: Brenner B, Coe FL, Rector FC, Jr, eds. Renal physiology in health and disease. Philadelphia: W.B. Saunders Company, 1987:112–131.

Levenson DJ. Structure and function of the renal circulations. In: Brenner B, Coe FL, Rector FC Jr, eds. Renal physiology in health and disease. Philadelphia: W.B. Saunders Company, 1987:1–16.

Rose BD. Clinical physiology of acid-base and electrolyte disorders. 2nd ed. Part 1. Water and electrolyte physiology. Part 2. Renal physiology. Part 3. Regulation of water and electrolyte balance. New York: McGraw-Hill Book Company, 1984:3–268.

NORMAL PHYSIOLOGY PROBLEMS

1. Estimate the pH from the following H^+ concentrations:
   A. 60 nEq/L   B. 34 nEq/L   C. 53 nEq/L

2. A patient has a GFR of 100 cc/min. What is the clearance of the substances in Column A. Select answers from Column B.

Column A	Column B
1. Urea (MW 60)	a. >100 cc/min
2. Creatinine (MW113)	b. 100 cc/min
3. Inulin (MW 5200)	c. <100 cc/min but >40 cc/min
4. Myoglobin (MW 17,000)	
5. Albumin (MW 69,000)	d. <10 cc/min

3. A. Your patient is a 20-year-old body builder. He is quite muscular and weighs 200 lbs. His Scr is 1.5 mg/dl. His 24-hour urine specimen contains 1400 ml and has a creatinine concentration of 70 mg/dl. How many mg of creatinine are in the specimen?

   B. What is the creatinine clearance in L/day?

   C. In mL/min?

   D. Is this a complete urine specimen?

N.B. mg/dl = mg/100 ml.

4. A. A 6-year-old child with a body surface area of 1 M^2 submits a 12-hour urine collection with 400 mg of creatinine. The Scr is 0.8 mg/dl. Calculate the creatinine clearance in ml/min.
   B. Correct the creatinine clearance to 1.73 M^2 body surface area. Is this normal?

5. A patient has a new renal transplant. He has had a stable Scr of 0.6 mg/dl. Six months after the transplant the level rises to 1.2 mg/dl. This change is most likely due to:
   a. a significant loss of GFR
   b. The normal daily fluctuation of Scr within the normal range
   c. A rise in creatinine production
   d. Impairment of protein synthesis due to corticosteroids

6. A. A patient develops azotemia with a Scr of 2.0 mg/dl and a BUN of 60 mg/dl. Two days later Scr and BUN are still 2.0 and 60 mg/dl, respectively. If a 24-hour urine shows increased urea excretion, name two possible causes:
   B. If the 24-hour urine shows normal urea excretion, name two possible causes:

7. A man weighs 220 lbs.
   A. What is his total body water?
   B. His extracellular volume?
   C. His intravascular volume?
   D. The man has a serum sodium concentration of 140 mEq/L and a plasma osmolality of 280 mOsm/kg. He drinks 3 L of beer over 10 min in a beer drinking contest. (The electrolyte content of beer is negligible) What is the plasma osmolality after this beer is absorbed, but before it is excreted by the kidneys?
   E. What is the serum sodium concentration?

8. Match the history in each case in Column A with the results of a 24-hour urine collection in Column B.

Column A	Column B
1. Normal man ingesting 150 mEq/day Na^+	a. 1 mEq Na^+/day
2. Man ingesting 150 mEq/day Na^+ with 3 L diarrhea (has 80 mEq Na^+/L)/day	b. 150 mEq Na^+/day
3. Man cheating on 150 mEq/day Na^+ restriction	c. 200 mEq Na^+/day
4. Man ingesting 150 mEq Na^+/day and 10 L water/day	d. 75 mEq Na^+/day

9. The drug acetazolamide inhibits proximal tubule carbonic anhydrase. In a patient taking this drug, will you see an increase, a decrease, or no change in proximal tubule reabsorption of HCO_3^-_____; of Na^+_____; of H_2O_____.

10. A 70-kg student with a plasma osmolality of 285 mOsm/kg begins to protest a recent tuition raise by refusing to eat or drink water.

   A. Within less than a day his urine will become maximally concentrated and his overall water loss from all sources will go down to about_____ml/day.

   B. About how much weight (in kg) would he lose from dehydration alone per day? (Disregard weight loss from utilization of fat stores.)

   C. Assuming no loss of total osmotic particles in the body and continued negative water balance at the same rate, what will plasma osmolality be after 2 days without water?

   D. What would this student's daily urinary losses of Na^+, HCO_3^-, and K^+ be once maximum urine conservation has been achieved?

   E. About what percent of total fluid compartment content of water, Na^+, and K^+ would be lost after 10 days of fasting? Select an answer from the following: >20%, 1–10%, 0.1–1%, ~0%.

11. A vegetarian ingests about 40 mEq of alkali equivalent per day. A 24-hour urine specimen would contain about:
    a. 40 mEq HCO_3^-
    b. 40 mEq free OH^-
    c. 40 mEq $H_2PO_4^-$
    d. 40 mEq NH_4^+
    e. 40 mEq free H^+

12. A. A patient ingests about 200 mEq of acid equivalent per day. A 24-hour urine specimen would contain:

mEq/day

	HCO_3^-	H_2PO_4	NH_4^+	H^+
a.	<1	40	40	120
b.	200	<1	<1	<1
c.	<1	160	40	<1
d.	<1	<1	<1	200
e.	<1	40	160	<1

   B. If the patient has a serum HCO_3^- concentration of 24 mEq/L and a GFR of 100 ml/min, how much total H^+ must be secreted by the tubules in a day to reabsorb all filtered HCO_3^-?
   C. How much total H^+ must be secreted by the tubules in a day to excrete the daily 200 mEq acid load?

13. Which of the following stimuli will increase ADH release.
    a. Increased BUN concentration
    b. Decreased BUN concentration
    c. Increased circulating volume
    d. Decreased circulating volume
    e. Decreased serum Na^+ concentration

14. A. A man on a normal diet, begins a low salt, normal K^+ diet. Match the items in Column A with one of the three possible answers in Column B.

Column A
1. Aldosterone level
2. Proximal tubular Na^+ reabsorption
3. Proximal tubule water reabsorption
4. Sodium delivery to the distal nephron
5. Water delivery to the distal nephron

Column B
a. Increases
b. Decreases
c. No change

B. You know that aldosterone stimulates K^+ secretion. However, normally, a low salt diet has no effect on K^+ excretion or serum K^+ level. How might you explain the failure of low salt diets to produce a K^+ deficit?
a. Sodium delivery to the K^+ secretion site is increased.
b. Sodium delivery to the K^+ secretion site is reduced.
c. Proximal K^+ reabsorption is increased.
d. Proximal K^+ reabsorption is decreased.
e. Aldosterone antagonizing hormone is released.

chapter 2

Volume Disorders

J. Gary Abuelo

Normal cardiac output and perfusion of the body's organs require normal cardiac filling pressure, which in turn depends on having normal intravascular volume. Overload (**hypervolemia**) and depletion (**hypovolemia**) of the intravascular volume are common in clinical medicine and may be seen in a variety of renal and extrarenal conditions. The causes and clinical consequences of these derangements will be discussed in this chapter. Since the interstitial volume usually expands and contracts with the intravascular volume, clinical swelling of the interstitial space, called **edema,** usually accompanies hypervolemia. Edema may also be seen with normal intravascular volume. The edematous states will also be covered in this chapter.

Hypervolemia

Etiology

Hypervolemia is an excess of intravascular volume. It could theoretically be caused by increased red cell volume, but, in fact, such cases are rare and limited to patients who have accidentally received excessive red cell transfusions. In clinical practice, excessive intravascular volume is almost always due to **increased plasma volume,** which in turn usually comes about through expansion of the extracellular space

Table 2.1.
Principal Causes of Hypervolemia

I. Increased red blood cell volume (excessive transfusion of packed cells)
II. Increased plasma volume
   A. Inadequate renal excretion of Na^+
     1. Heart failure
     2. Primary renal Na^+ retention
       a. Renal failure
       b. Primary mineralocorticoid excess, e.g. primary aldosteronism
       c. Inhibition of prostaglandin synthesis (NSAID)[a]
   B. Massive intake of Na^+

---

[a]NSAID—nonsteroidal anti-inflammatory drugs.

secondary to **inadequate renal excretion of Na^+** (Table 2.1). Extracellular volume increases when the body accumulates water isotonically with the Na^+ in order to maintain normal osmolarity. Massive oral or intravenous intake of salt can overwhelm the normal kidney's Na^+ excreting ability; however, given the kidney's large natriuretic capacity, this is a rare clinical event and will not be discussed further.

Pathogenesis

Heart Failure

Heart failure or cardiac output inadequate for the needs of the body is the most common cause of hypervolemia in clinical medicine. Initially, the hypervolemia may increase atrial filling and partially restore cardiac output toward normal. However, with worsening of heart disease, more fluid can accumulate and produce serious symptoms. Indeed, the major manifestations of heart failure are the "congestive changes" caused by hypervolemia.

Inadequate cardiac output produces hypervolemia by stimulating renal Na^+ retention, i.e. reducing Na^+ excretion. The body simultaneously retains water to maintain normal tonicity. Multiple mechanisms of renal Na^+ retention are recognized, but the relative importance of each is not known. They involve both a decrease in glomerular filtration of Na^+ and an increase in tubular reabsorption (Fig. 2.1). Decreased filtration of Na^+ occurs when reduced cardiac output leads to lower blood pressure, thus decreasing renal perfusion and, in turn, GFR. Increased tubular reabsorption of Na^+ is the culmination of a series of events, which begin when the body's baroreceptors sense

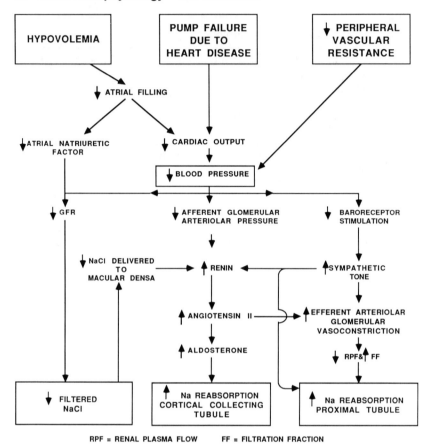

RPF = RENAL PLASMA FLOW   FF = FILTRATION FRACTION

Figure 2.1. Mechanisms of renal sodium conservation in response to heart failure and other types of decreased effective blood volume.

reduced cardiac output and blood pressure. It is said that they detect decreased **effective blood volume.** This term is an attempt to reconcile the facts that hypervolemia is present in heart failure, but the barore-ceptors' response is typical of hypovolemia, presumably because the blood volume is not effective in maintaining organ perfusion. It may be that the baroreceptors mainly respond to arterial volume, which would be reduced by a fall in either peripheral resistance or cardiac output. Unfortunately, no instrument can measure volume circulating **effectively** or occupying the arterial tree, so effective blood volume cannot be measured or even defined very precisely. Three mechanisms of increased tubular reabsorption of Na^+ have been described as follows.

Sympathetic Stimulation of the Proximal Tubule. Vasomotor centers in the brain stem increase sympathetic neural tone in response to a fall in signals from the arterial baroreceptors. Sympathetic stimulation via systemic and local release of norepinephrine increases renin secretion and may directly stimulate proximal tubular reabsorption of Na^+.

Aldosterone Stimulation of the Cortical Collecting Tubule. **Increased renin secretion** may be a response to three stimuli: 1) decreased perfusion of the afferent glomerular arterioles which have baroreceptors, 2) decreased NaCl delivery to the macula densa in the distal tubule, and 3) increased sympathetic tone. Renin secretion via activation of angiotensin leads to increased aldosterone levels, which in turn cause Na^+ reabsorption in the cortical collecting tubule.

Starling Forces Acting on the Peritubular Capillaries. Angiotensin and sympathetic stimulation via norepinephrine **increase resistance in the efferent glomerular arterioles** in order to maintain hydrostatic pressure in the glomerular capillaries. This preserves GFR, while it increases total renal resistance and reduces renal blood flow. Since less renal plasma flow yields the same amount of glomerular filtrate, the fraction of blood filtered across the glomerular capillary walls (or **filtration fraction**) is higher. As a consequence of these changes, the blood coming out of the glomeruli into the peritubular capillaries has a lower hydrostatic pressure and a higher protein concentration, both of which alter Starling forces in favor of fluid uptake by the capillaries. This in turn **increases Na^+ reabsorption by the proximal tubules.** The various mechanisms by which decreased circulating effective volume leads to renal Na^+ retention are depicted in Figure 2.1.

Renal Failure

This is a common cause of hypervolemia. The level of GFR at which volume overload is seen varies, but generally is less than 10–20 ml/min and corresponds to a Scr greater than 5 mg/dl. The kidney's ability to maintain Na^+ homeostasis in the face of an 80% or greater loss of GFR is due to its large reserve capacity to eliminate Na^+. The kidney normally filters over 100 times the Na^+ excreted and then **must do work** to reabsorb more than 99% of it. If the GFR falls to one-tenth of normal, the kidney filters only about 10 times the Na^+ it must excrete and just reabsorbs about 90% of it (Fig. 2.2). This reduction in percent

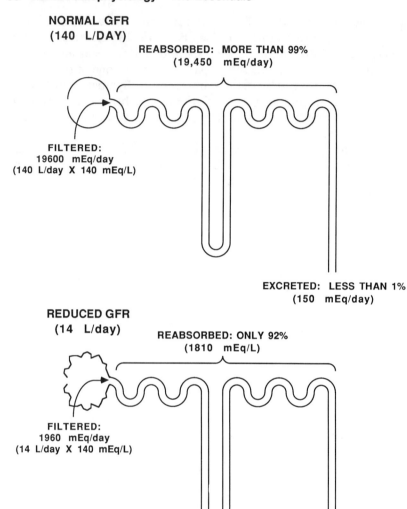

NORMAL GFR
(140 L/DAY)

REABSORBED: MORE THAN 99%
(19,450   mEq/day)

FILTERED:
19600 mEq/day
(140 L/day X 140 mEq/L)

EXCRETED: LESS THAN 1%
(150   mEq/day)

REDUCED GFR
(14 L/day)

REABSORBED: ONLY 92%
(1810   mEq/L)

FILTERED:
1960 mEq/day
(14 L/day X 140 mEq/L)

EXCRETED: ABOUT 8%
(150   mEq/day)

Figure 2.2. Maintenance of Na$^+$ excretion through reduced tubular reabsorption in the face of a 90% loss of GFR.

Na^+ reabsorption from over 99 to about 90%, as GFR falls, protects most patients from hypervolemia, which is only seen with further loss of GFR.

Primary Mineralocorticoid Excess

Adrenal adenomas that produce excessive amounts of aldosterone may induce renal Na^+ retention. The aldosterone stimulates Na^+ reabsorption in the cortical collecting tubule. The degree of hypervolemia is limited, however, and edema formation is usually not seen. This limitation is due to the "escape phenomenon," which is presumably caused by compensatory changes in the body's other mechanisms for maintaining euvolemia through the control of Na^+ excretion. Thus, aldosterone induced Na^+ retention is counterbalanced by atrial natriuretic factor, GFR, renin, angiotensin and sympathetic tone, all of which respond to the hypervolemia by increasing filtered Na^+ and reducing proximal reabsorption of Na^+.

Nonsteroidal Anti-Inflammatory Drugs (NSAID)

NSAID such as indomethacin can also produce Na^+ retention. These drugs are used commonly to treat arthritis and inhibit renal synthesis of prostaglandins. Under conditions of decreased effective circulating volume, such as congestive heart failure or volume depletion, these hormones or autocoids tend to maintain renal Na^+ excretion. The site of this natriuretic action of prostaglandins is not known. Occasionally, the administration of NSAID to patients with mild congestive heart failure causes hypervolemia, which is thought to be mediated by this inhibition of prostaglandin synthesis. NSAID has also produced hypervolemia in patients without a known predisposing factor, presumably mediated by reduced prostaglandin production.

Clinical Features

Because of their high compliance, any increase in intravascular volume is mainly distributed to the veins, increasing venous and right and left atrial pressures. In the heart increased filling pressure leads to increased end diastolic volume and augmented cardiac output. The arterial blood pressure rises, due to this relationship: **arterial pressure = cardiac output × peripheral vascular resistance.** The high venous pressure is also transmitted to the capillary bed, where the high hydrostatic pressure increases filtration of fluid into the interstitium due to the change in Starling forces.

When intravascular volume expansion exceeds about 10%, venous engorgement can be seen as distended neck veins or hepatomegaly on physical examination and as pulmonary vascular congestion on chest x-ray. The distended heart may manifest tachycardia, murmurs and a gallop rhythm. The chest x-ray may also show the increased cardiac volume as cardiomegaly. Blood pressure often rises and severe hypertension may develop. In patients with heart failure, however, cardiac output is reduced and hypertension, if seen, is caused by catecholamine induced peripheral vasoconstriction.

Initially, as increased fluid filters from the capillaries, the rise in interstitial pressure increases lymphatic flow, which drains off the excess fluid. With greater movement of fluid into the interstitium **edema** (clinically apparent swelling of this fluid compartment) forms mainly in dependent areas of the body and in the pulmonary interstitium. This gives rise to ankle swelling, orthopnea, dyspnea on exertion and basilar rales. With progressive retention of salt and water the edema may become generalized (anasarca), extending to the torso and face. With anasarca, accumulation of edema fluid in the peritoneal space (ascites) and in the pleural space (hydrothorax) may be seen. Pulmonary and peripheral edema tend to occur more or less simultaneously in many patients. In some cases, however, either pulmonary or peripheral edema presents alone, with the other occurring later or not at all. The reason for this is clear in patients with hypervolemia due to predominantly left- or right-sided heart failure. There is no obvious reason in other cases.

Although hypervolemia is caused by excess accumulation of Na^+, serum Na^+ levels are usually normal, owing to the body's maintenance of tonicity. Occasionally (see chapter on **tonicity disorders**) more water accumulates than is needed to achieve isotonicity, which **lowers serum Na^+ concentration below normal.** Despite this **hyponatremia,** these hypervolemic patients, nevertheless, have **excessive total body Na^+ content.**

Diagnosis

Hypervolemia may be diagnosed when peripheral edema or pulmonary edema or both appear together with signs of increased venous filling, such as distended neck veins or pulmonary vascular congestion on chest x-ray. Additionally, one should see hypertension, tachycardia, cardiomegaly and an S3 gallop. Occasionally, a patient may have edema without other manifestations of hypervolemia (see section on **edematous states** below), and one may be uncertain of the volume status. If one needs to verify the hypervolemic status of such a patient, a Swan-Ganz (balloon tip) catheter may be passed through a peripheral vein into the heart, where it can measure right atrial pressure. It may also be placed in a small pulmonary artery where the small balloon cuts off blood flow. The pressure measured under these circumstances is that transmitted from the left atrium. The right and left atrial pressures so measured accurately characterize cardiac filling pressures. The peripheral vascular resistance and cardiac output may also be determined.

One may diagnose renal insufficiency as the cause of hypervolemia from an elevated Scr, usually >5 mg/dl. Aldosterone-producing tumors typically cause hypertension, and little, if any edema. Aldosterone causes increased tubular secretion of H^+ and K^+, so that metabolic alkalosis and hypokalemia (see chapters on **acid-base disorders** and **potassium disorders**) should suggest this diagnosis, which may be confirmed by demonstrating high plasma aldosterone levels. The role of NSAID in causing hypervolemia is best confirmed by stopping the suspected medication and observing improvement in the volume overload. Heart failure is the most common cause of hypervolemia and is the first diagnosis that should come to mind. It often is accompanied by other evidence of heart disease such as murmurs, angina pectoris, myocardial infarction or arrhythmias. Generally, since other causes of hypervolemia may simulate heart failure, a diagnosis of heart failure should be made only after other causes have been excluded.

Treatment

In some cases the primary cause of hypervolemia may be treated: renal failure may be improved; adrenal adenomas may be surgically removed; NSAID may be stopped; defective heart valves may be replaced; and cardiac function may be improved with vasodilators or digitalis. More often the primary problem is intractable, and one uses dietary Na^+ restriction and diuretics to treat hypervolemia. As one reduces total body Na^+ to normal, the body will usually excrete water to avoid hypotonicity. Therefore, water restriction is usually unnecessary.

Hypovolemia

Etiology

Hypovolemia is depletion of intravascular volume. It may involve either loss of whole blood during hemorrhage or loss of plasma volume without red cells due to fluid depletion from the extracellular space through any one of several routes (Table 2.2). We shall see below that hypovolemia occurs with Na^+ and water loss, but is usually negligible with water loss alone. Thus, depletion of total body Na^+ is almost a sine qua non for hypovolemia.

Pathogenesis

Loss of body fluids does not always produce volume depletion. Slow bleeding, such as menstruation, can be replenished by increased erythropoiesis and production of plasma proteins, just as slow fluid loss, such as from mild diarrhea, can be replenished by reduced renal excre-

Table 2.2.
Principal Causes of Hypovolemia

I.   Whole blood loss (hemorrhage from any site)
II. Plasma loss
    A. Renal losses of Na^+ and water
        1. Osmotic diuresis, e.g. glycosuria 2° diabetes mellitus
        2. Diuretics
        3. Aldosterone deficiency, e.g. primary adrenal insufficiency
        4. Diabetes insipidus
    B. Extrarenal losses Na^+ and water
        1. Gastrointestinal fluid
            a. Vomiting, drainage from nasogastric tube
            b. Biliary or pancreatic drainage tubes
            c. Fistula
            d. Diarrhea
        2. Skin losses
            a. Sweating
            b. Weeping from burns
            c. Insensible loss due to fever or hot environment
        3. Sequestration into interstitial or transcellular space ("third spacing")
            a. Crushed limb
            b. Intestinal obstruction

tion of dietary Na^+ and water, which are usually ingested in amounts far in excess of basal needs. Thus, the pathogenesis of hypovolemia generally requires moderate-to-severe loss of blood or body fluids.

Role of Composition of Lost Fluids

The impact of fluid loss on intravascular volume depends on the composition of the lost fluid. Whole blood loss has the greatest impact, since it comes directly from the vascular space. It should be noted that the volume loss lowers venous pressure and in turn capillary hydrostatic pressure. The change in Starling forces reduces or stops filtration of fluid out of the capillaries. This leads to partial restitution of blood volume from the interstitial space, as the direction of net filtration reverses into the capillaries and as the lymphatics return fluid to the vascular bed. The proportion of red cell volume to plasma volume (hematocrit) is unchanged in the vascular compartment immediately following blood loss, but will fall over several hours as the red cells are diluted by refilling of the vascular space from the interstitium.

Loss of isotonic fluid leads to depletion of the extracellular space, of which one-fourth is in the intravascular volume. Therefore, one might expect that about one-fourth of lost isotonic fluid might come from the plasma portion of the intravascular compartment. The actual contribution of plasma volume to the loss is probably even less than this, since fluid loss from the plasma increases the protein concentration (oncotic pressure). Also capillary hydrostatic pressure falls, so that filtration of fluid from the capillaries slows. As a result, there is a tendency of extracellular fluid to shift into the intravascular compartment, leading to a disproportionate loss from the interstitial space and relative protection of the plasma volume.

Relatively pure water loss occurs in certain clinical situations, such as the patient with high insensible loss due to fever. When water without solutes is lost from the body, it comes from both intracellular and extracellular spaces, which maintain equal osmolarity to one another. About 10% of body water is in plasma and red cells in the intravascular space; therefore, **no more than one-tenth** of lost body water comes from the vascular compartment. Because of the rise in plasma oncotic pressure that occurs with volume depletion, the impact of pure water loss from the body on blood volume may be even smaller than this. Thus, there is little reduction of intravascular volume from pure water loss and it is unusual to see clinically significant hypovolemia. This has led to the clinical maxim that **Na^+ depletion is necessary to have volume**

depletion. Thus, although a patient with hypertonicity due to water loss will have an **increased serum Na$^+$ concentration,** if he has volume depletion, it means that Na$^+$ has also been lost and **total body Na$^+$ is reduced.**

Regulation of Tonicity

The body fluids that may be lost in the hypovolemic states include urine, sweat and fluids from the gut. From Table 2.3, we see that many of these fluids are hypotonic.

Nevertheless, most patients with fluid loss from the body maintain normal tonicity. In some cases, this is because of the isotonic nature of the fluid lost (e.g. "third spacing" or loss of bile post operatively from a drainage tube). In other cases, stimulation of thirst and elaboration of a concentrated urine lead to replenishment of the excess water lost in hypotonic fluids.

Renal Fluid Losses

Renal fluid losses may occur through four mechanisms. First, there may be an increased filtered load of osmotically active particles, such as glucose in diabetes mellitus, which retain water and Na$^+$ in the tubular lumen and greatly increase urine losses (osmotic diuresis; see polyuria in chapter on **tonicity disorders**). Second, diuretics impair tubular Na$^+$ reabsorption and increase both urine Na$^+$ and water loss.

Table 2.3.
Approximate Electrolyte Composition of
Several Body Fluids

	Electrolyte Composition (mEq/L)			
	Na$^+$	K$^+$	Cl$^-$	HCO$_3^-$
Urine[a]	<80	50	80	0
Sweat	50	5	50	0
Gastric juice	50	10	90	0
Bile, ileal fluid	140	10	80	30
Pancreatic fluid	140	10	70	80
Diarrheal fluid	80	30	70	30

[a]Variable, depending on Na$^+$ intake, intravascular volume or use of diuretics.

Third, adrenal disease may impair aldosterone secretion and, in turn, decrease reabsorption of Na^+ in the cortical collecting duct. Fourth, several conditions may impair renal water reabsorption in the distal nephron, leading to loss of large volumes of dilute urine, i.e. diabetes insipidus (see next chapter on **tonicity disorders**).

Clinical Features

The amount of blood withdrawn during blood donation is 500 cc, which is about 10% of the blood volume. This reduces venous return to the heart and tends to lower stroke volume, cardiac output and blood pressure. However, sympathetic activity increases heart rate, mitigating the loss of cardiac output. In addition, arteriolar vasoconstriction from increased sympathetic activity and activation of the renin angiotensin system increases peripheral resistance, thus maintaing normal blood pressure:

Normal arterial pressure = Normal cardiac output

$\times$ normal resistance

Normal arterial pressure = **Low** cardiac output $\times$ **high** resistance

The blood donor is, therefore, usually asymptomatic, although his kidneys will respond to the mild hypovolemia by reducing Na^+ excretion (Fig. 2.1).

Greater degrees of intravascular volume loss ($>15\%$ blood volume) produce hypotension, which first appears in the upright position as a sensation of faintness or actual loss of consciousness (fainting, syncope). The patient may notice a greying or blackening of the vision, giving rise to the term "blackout." Sitting or lying improves venous return and consciousness returns. The patient may be thirsty or may have muscle cramps.

Physical examination shows a low blood pressure and tachycardia, although initially these are only seen when the patient is seated or standing. The mouth and skin, including the axillae, are dry. The elasticity of the skin is lost, so that a pinch of skin remains "tented" for a while, instead of flattening immediately. One may see no filling of the external jugular veins on laying the patient flat.

Severe hypovolemia may precipitate **shock,** in which low cardiac output and peripheral vessels vasoconstricted by high sympathetic activity reduce tissue perfusion. There is inadequate delivery to cells of nutrients and oxygen and inadequate removal of wastes and CO_2. This results in abnormal anaerobic cellular metabolism, which, if unchecked, can lead to cell death. Poor renal perfusion reduces GFR, resulting in azotemia. Urine flow falls and urine is concentrated due to reduced glomerular filtration of water and high ADH secretion in response to hypovolemia. Volume (Na^+) regulatory mechanisms reduce renal Na^+ excretion (Fig. 2.1). Therefore, despite high urine concentration, urine Na^+ concentration is low (<10 mEq/L) unless the hypovolemia is caused by renal Na^+ losing. Thus, shock is characterized clinically by hypotension, tachycardia, vasoconstricted extremities (cold, clammy, cyanotic), confusion, azotemia and a low output of concentrated Na^+-poor urine.

Despite the fact that hypovolemia is frequently due to loss of hypotonic body fluids, thanks to the body's maintenance of normal tonicity, serum Na^+ concentration and plasma osmolality are usually normal. However, sometimes these mechanisms fail and either hyper- or hyponatremia are seen. This is discussed in the chapter on **tonicity disorders.**

Diagnosis

Hypovolemia reduces cardiac output and lowers blood pressure. The absence of edema and increased venous filling in hypovolemia distinguishes it from reduced cardiac output and low blood pressure seen in **cardiac pump failure** produced, for example, by a severe myocardial infarction. (There are no edema, distended neck veins, hepatomegaly or pulmonary vascular congestion in hypovolemia). Hypovolemia must also be distinguished from the low blood pressure seen with decreased peripheral resistance due to **sepsis** or excessive **antihypertensive medications,** which would be suggested by a fever or the drug history, respectively. If a question exists as to the mechanism of hypotension, measurement of the left atrial pressure, cardiac output and peripheral resistance through a Swan-Ganz catheter might be needed.

The source of fluid loss in volume depletion is usually obvious from the history. If no fluid losses have been noted, a determination of urine Na^+ concentration may be helpful. A value of <10 mEq/L would demonstrate a normal renal response to hypovolemia and would suggest some occult extrarenal loss, such as third spacing or internal bleeding. Surreptitious vomiting or laxative abuse should also be considered despite vigorous denial in persons attempting to lose weight, such as competitive wrestlers or women with anorexia nervosa. A urine Na^+ concentration of >20 mEq/L would be inappropriately high in a volume-depleted patient and would suggest that the source of Na^+ loss is the urine itself; diuretics or aldosterone deficiency would be possible causes.

Treatment

The cause of the fluid loss should be treated if possible. The current volume deficit should be estimated and replaced. The rate of fluid loss should be estimated and oral or intravenous maintenance fluids should be provided.

In general there are three types of intravenous fluids: 1) whole blood (or separated red cells and plasma), 2) normal or isotonic saline (154 mEq/L NaCl), and 3) isotonic 5% dextrose in water (D5W; the dextrose is metabolised in the body, leaving free water). In general, blood loss is replaced with blood and extracellular volume deficit is replaced with normal saline. Mixtures of D5W and normal saline are used as maintenance fluids to prevent further deficits in patients unable to take fluids by mouth. For example, 1000 cc of urine with 77 mEq/L NaCl would be the equivalent of 500 cc normal saline and 500 cc D5W. Insensible losses contain no electrolytes and are replaced with D5W.

Edematous States

Edema or swelling of the interstitial space with fluid may involve the lungs or the periphery. In the periphery edema may be local (e.g. a "black eye") or generalized.

Etiology

Although edema is often due to hypervolemia, the physician must also consider other causes, the most important of which are listed in Table 2.4.

Pathogenesis

Edema or tissue swelling is due to a local increase in the volume of the interstitial space. It may be produced by increased filtration of fluid

Table 2.4.
Principal Causes of Edema[a]

I.   Increased capillary hydrostatic pressure
   A. Hypervolemia (increased plasma volume)
      1. Inadequate renal excretion of Na^+
         a. Heart failure
         b. Primary renal Na^+ retention
            i. Renal failure
            ii. Inhibition of prostaglandins synthesis (NSAID)
      2. Massive intake of Na^+
   B. Venous obstruction or stasis
      1. Thrombosis
      2. Tumor compression
      3. Muscle disuse
      4. Tense ascites (liver disease)
II. Decreased plasma oncotic pressure due to hypoalbuminemia
   A. Reduced albumin synthesis
      1. Liver disease
      2. Malnutrition
   B. Urinary protein loss (nephrotic syndrome)
III. Increased capillary permeability
   A. Inflammation
   B. Trauma
   C. Burns
IV. Lymphatic obstruction (lymphedema) e.g. tumor

---

[a]Modified from Rose BD. Clinical physiology of acid-base and electrolyte disorders. 2nd ed. New York: McGraw-Hill Book Company, 1984:314.

across the capillary wall or by decreased lymphatic return of the fluid to the venous system.

Increased Capillary Hydrostatic Pressure

In the hypervolemic states elevated venous pressure may be transmitted to the capillary bed and produce edema, especially of dependent parts of the body. Similarly, the veins of one lower extremity may become thrombosed or may develop stasis due to lack of muscular pumping action and the resulting rise in intracapillary pressure will produce unilateral edema. Also tense ascites in patients with cirrhosis can partly occlude the inferior vena cava, raising venous pressure in the lower extremities.

Hypoalbuminemia

When serum albumin falls below 3 gm/dl (normal 4–5 gm/dl) due to reduced hepatic albumin synthesis, malnutrition or urinary protein loss (nephrotic syndrome; see chapter on **glomerular disorders**), the drop in plasma oncotic pressure leads to a high rate of fluid filtration across the capillary wall and edema formation. The lungs, however, do not develop edema with hypoalbuminemia. The pulmonary capillaries normally are permeable to albumin. Thus, interstitial albumin levels in the lung are rather high and the oncotic pressure difference between plasma and interstitium is small (Table 2.5), as is the pulmonary capillary hydrostatic pressure. When serum albumin levels fall, similar falls occur in interstitial albumin levels. Consequently, the oncotic pressure difference across the pulmonary capillary wall drops insignificantly and the rate of fluid escape only increases slightly.

Increased Capillary Permeability

Any local injury or inflammatory process may increase capillary permeability due to release of mediators from injured tissue, platelets and inflammatory cells. Loss of protein from the capillaries raises interstitial oncotic pressure, which, together with greater capillary wall permeability, increases the outward passage of fluid and causes local edema.

Table 2.5.
Capillary and Interstitial Oncotic Pressures (mm Hg) in the Pulmonary Circulation Compared to Those in the Peripheral Circulation[a]

	Pulmonary	Skeletal Muscle
Capillary	26	26
Interstitial	16	5.3
Difference	10	20.7

[a]Modified from Rose BD. Clinical physiology of acid-base and electrolyte disorders. 2nd ed. New York: McGraw-Hill Book Company, 1984:304.

Lymphatic Blockage

Finally, neoplastic diseases, like lymphomas, that invade the lymphatics and lymph nodes may produce local edema by blocking lymphatic return.

Role of Reduced Renal Excretion of Salt and Water in Edema Formation

The amount of edema formed may vary from miniscule (swollen lip from trauma) to massive. Generally, one needs about 3 L of edema fluid before generalized edema is detectable on examination and patients with nephrotic syndrome may gain 30 kg or more in edema fluid! Clearly, the generation of generalized edema requires more than a shift of fluid out of the vascular compartment, since a shift of 700 cc or more would cause hypovolemia or even shock. Also the resulting fall in intravascular volume would reduce venous and capillary hydrostatic pressure, thereby inhibiting further filtration of fluid out of the capillary. What actually happens in the edematous states is that at the same time as fluid leaves the capillary bed, the kidney retains dietary Na^+. To maintain isotonicity, the kidney also retains water, which refills the intravascular space. Over many weeks to months, massive edema may accumulate equivalent in extreme cases to one month's entire intake of salt.

Renal Na^+ retention may initiate the edema formation or may be a response to the edema formation (Fig. 2.3). In cases with hypervolemia, inadequate renal Na^+ excretion itself causes and maintains the high intravascular volume that leads to edema formation. In all of the other forms of edema, such as local venous obstruction, the loss of fluid from the capillary bed slightly decreases circulating volume. This stimulates secondary renal Na^+ retention. If the edema formation is gradual and there is ample Na^+ in the diet, renal retention of Na^+ will refill and prevent any depletion of the intravascular volume. These edema forming states are, therefore, marked by low normal intravascular volume.

Clinical Features

Peripheral edema is swelling that can pit. That is, prolonged pressure with a finger will force fluid out and leave a depression in the skin and subcutaneous tissue that lasts for several minutes. This will distinguish

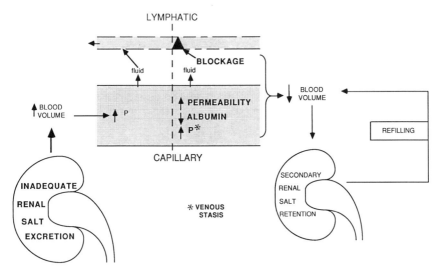

Figure 2.3.   Depiction of edema formation at the capillary level. On the *left side* of the diagram, edema results from inadequate renal salt excretion and hypervolemia as seen in heart or renal failure. On the *right side* of the diagram low serum albumin or a local factor like venous obstruction causes fluid to leave the circulatory bed, reducing blood volume. Secondary renal salt retention acts to refill the vascular tree.

edema from fat or infiltration by tumor. Typically edema first appears in dependent areas, where capillary hydrostatic pressure is greatest. Thus, swelling occurs in the feet and ankles during the day after sitting and standing and shifts to the back (sacral edema) and sometimes the face after the patient spends the night in a recumbent position. With worsening peripheral edema the lower extremities become tensely swollen with only slight improvement during the night, edema extends to the torso, and ascites and hydrothorax may occur. Thus, pleural effusions can be seen with the nephrotic syndrome in the absence of pulmonary edema.

Normal individuals may form edema of the lower extremities after standing for long periods, especially in warm weather. This is a result of reduced muscle activity, which normally pumps blood up the veins and keeps venous pressure low. This type of edema can also be seen in an arm or leg that has been immobilized by a cast or paralysis.

Pulmonary edema reduces gas exchange, particularly of oxygen, and produces dyspnea on effort, orthopnea and paroxysmal nocturnal dyspnea. Physical examination shows basilar rales and the chest x-ray shows the edematous (congested) lungs.

Despite the fact that edema formation involves the accumulation of excess Na^+ in the body, serum Na^+ concentrations are usually **normal** due to the body's effectiveness in maintaining normal tonicity through the stimulation of thirst and production of a concentrated urine.

Diagnosis

The physical examination will reveal whether the edema is a local process or is generalized. If the edema is localized, one should look for local causes such as venous or lymphatic obstruction. Venous obstruction may appear as dilated cutaneous veins in the involved area. Enlarged lymph nodes may be noted on physical examination. In patients with local edema, one may do a venogram or lymphangiogram, which are x-rays with contrast media injected into the veins or lymphatics to be examined, in order to confirm the diagnosis. If edema is caused by hypervolemia, the patient will usually demonstrate typical physical signs (hypertension, distended neck veins, rales, gallop and hepatomegaly). An elevated Scr will distinguish renal insufficiency from heart failure. Hypoalbuminemic states can be diagnosed by measuring a serum albumin level. Patients with the nephrotic syndrome will have large amounts of protein in the urine.

Treatment

The primary disease should be treated, if possible. If not, edema may be controlled nonspecifically by several means. Elevation of the lower extremities or elastic stocking can reduce intracapillary hydrostatic pressure or facilitate lymphatic return. Policemen, sales clerks and others who stand all day in their jobs often use such support stockings. A low-salt diet and diuretics will reduce total body Na^+, intravascular volume and capillary hydrostatic pressure. Filtration of fluid out of the capillaries will be inhibited, and edema may be completely reabsorbed in many cases. Hypovolemia and hypotension can be a complication of this therapy.

Suggested Readings

Abboud FM. Shock. In: Wyngaarden JB, Smith LH, Jr., eds. Cecil textbook of medicine. Philadelphia: W.B. Saunders Company, 1988:236–250.

Andreoli TE. Disorders of fluid volume, electrolyte, and acid-base balance. In: Wyngaarden JB, Smith LH, Jr., eds. Cecil textbook of medicine. Philadelphia: W.B. Saunders Company, 1988:528–536.

Hollenberg NK. The kidney in heart failure. Hospital Practice 1986;21:81–100.

Rose BD. Clinical physiology of acid-base and electrolyte disorders. 2nd ed. Regulation of the effective circulating volume (Chap. 9); Hypovolemic states (Chap. 15); Edematous states and the use of diuretics (Chap. 16). New York:McGraw-Hill Book Company, 1984:171–190, 279–360.

VOLUME DISORDER PROBLEMS

1. A 60-year-old woman with chronic renal insufficiency and anemia is admitted to the hospital for cosmetic surgery. The physical examination is normal; the Ccr is 10 ml/min; and the Scr is 4 mg/dl. In preparation for surgery the next day, the patient receives 500 ml of packed red cells and the intravenous line is kept open with 1 L of normal saline given over 24 hours. She has a ham steak for the evening meal. At 1 a.m. the patient develops pulmonary edema. All of the following factors probably contributed to the onset of pulmonary edema **EXCEPT:**
   a. Assuming a recumbent position
   b. Underlying renal insufficiency
   c. High Na^+ load
   d. Further deterioration of renal function
   e. Blood transfusions

2. In the patient with decreased effective circulating volume, increased sympathetic tone:
   a. suppresses renin secretion
   b. causes tachycardia
   c. lowers peripheral resistance
   d. dilates the efferent glomerular arterioles
   e. stimulates Na^+ reabsorption at the ascending loop of Henle

3. In the patient with congestive heart failure, increased filtration fraction:
   a. indirectly increases Na^+ reabsorption by the proximal tubule
   b. results in lower peritubular protein concentration
   c. is a consequence of reduced catecholamine and renin activity
   d. is associated with increased renal plasma flow
   e. is caused by reduced glomerular capillary hydrostatic pressure

4. A. Will renin secretion be increased or decreased in patients with high aldosterone levels caused by volume depletion? B. by adrenal adenoma?

5. Which of the following patients is most likely to have hypervolemia with increased total body Na^+?

	Pulmonary Edema + Vascular Congestion on X-ray	Jugular Venous Distention	Pleural Effusions	Peripheral Edema	Serum Albumin (gm/dl)	Serum Na (mEq/L)
a.	−	−	+	+	2.0	140
b.	−	−	−	−	4.0	160
c.	+	−	−	−	4.0	130
d.	−	−	−	+	4.0	140
e.	−	−	+	−	4.0	160

6. A 70-year-old man with longstanding angina pectoris and arthritis is admitted to the hospital with a 1-week history of worsening chest pain, ankle edema, dyspnea on effort and orthopnea. His normal blood pressure is 120/60 mm Hg. On physical examination you find blood pressure 140/90 mm Hg, pulse 100/min, distended jugular veins, bibasilar rales, an S3 gallop, a Grade III holosystolic murmur at the apex, hepatomegaly, and 2+ edema below the knees.

You might order all of the following tests. However, if you had to choose just **three** of these diagnostic steps, which would be most helpful in discovering the **cause** of your patient's condition?
   a. Chest X-ray
   b. Electrocardiogram and CPK levels
   c. Obtain a complete list of medications
   d. Serum Na^+ level
   e. Scr level
   f. Serum albumin level
   g. 24-hour urine for protein
7. A patient has hypovolemia with a 700-cc decrease in blood volume. Estimate the minimum volume of fluid you would have to give the patient to repair the deficit:
   A. if you were giving whole blood to replace blood loss
   B. if you were giving normal saline to replace extracellular depletion
   C. if you were giving D5W to replace pure water loss

8. A. A 20-year-old man develops food poisoning after eating out. For 12 hours he has repeated vomiting and profuse diarrhea and is unable to drink anything. He develops weakness and loss of vision on standing and is admitted to the hospital at midnight. Which of the following set of "numbers" would best fit this patient?

Recumbent Pulse and Blood Pressure (mm Hg)	Standing Pulse and Blood Pressure (mm Hg)	Hematocrit (Normally 40%)	Serum Na (mEq/L)	Urine	
				Na(mEq/L)	Osm/ kg
a. 80/min; 120/80	120/min; 80/50	47%	151	1	900
b. 80/min; 120/80	120/min; 80/50	47%	151	140	900
c. 120/min; 80/50	120/min; 80/50	40%	140	1	900
d. 120/min; 80/50	120/min; 80/50	47%	140	1	285
e. 80/min; 120/80	80/min; 120/80	40%	151	1	900

B. An intravenous infusion is started, but accidentally stops flowing almost immediately. At 8 a.m. the patient had 900 ml of diarrhea over 8 hours, but he has not vomited since admission and he is able to keep down fluids. His numbers now show:

80/min; 120/80   120/min; 80/50   47%   140   1   900

Explain how any difference between this set of numbers and the earlier set came about.

C. The patient weighs 4.4 lbs less than he did the morning before admission. Assuming this weight loss is all due to gastrointestinal fluid loss, what fluids would you have to give to replace his deficit—whole blood, normal saline, and/or D5W? How much would you give him?

D. You order the patient to have nothing by mouth, and order intravenous fluids to replace his deficit (from C. above). **In addition,** you order **maintenance** intravenous fluids to cover ongoing fluid loss for the next 24 hours. You may order either D5W or normal saline or some of each. Assuming that his diarrhea continues at the same rate, what volume of fluids would you order to cover.

	D5W	*Saline*
	(ml/24 hours)	*(ml/24 hours)*

Net extra renal loss from skin and respiratory
tract minus water of metabolism?
Renal loss?
GI loss?

9. A 50-year-old woman with a history of hypertension comes to the
hospital emergency room complaining that she is too weak to get
out of bed and has been thirsty. An examination with the patient
recumbent shows blood pressure 110/70 mm Hg, pulse 92/min,
and cool, slightly cyanotic extremities. Laboratory studies show
BUN 34 mg/dl, Scr 1.5 mg/dl, urine osmolality 930 mOsm/kg.

A. Diagnostic possibilities with this preliminary information
include all of the following **EXCEPT:**

   a. Adrenal insufficiency
   b. Silent myocardial infarction
   c. Overdose of antihypertensive medications
   d. Occult hemorrhage
   e. High protein diet

B. For each diagnostic possibility in Column A select the information in Column B which would support that particular
diagnosis:

Column A
1. Adrenal insufficiency
2. Silent myocardial infarction
3. Excessive vasodilatation from antihypertensive medication
4. Occult hemorrhage
5. High protein diet

Column B

	U_{Na}(mEq/L)	Cardiac Output	Neck Veins at 30°	Neck Veins of Patient Flat
a.	7	Decreased	Distended	Distended
b.	80	Normal	Flat	Distended
c.	7	Decreased	Flat	Flat
d.	80	Decreased	Flat	Flat
e.	7	Increased	Flat	Distended

C. The neck veins were flat with the patient lying flat. The patient had not increased her longstanding dose of antihypertensives. The patient denies vomiting, diarrhea or excessive sweating. The hematocrit is high normal. Give two diagnoses you might expect if the $U_{Na} = 3$ mEq/L:

if the $U_{Na} = 50$ mEq/L:

10. A. A 60-year-old schizophrenic man had two myocardial infarctions in the past. Two months ago he begins to sit immobile in a chair all day. He develops bilateral edema below the knees. There is no improvement with digoxin. The diagnosis might be suggested by any of the following pieces of information **EXCEPT:**

    a. Increase in weight over past 2 months

    b. Scrum albumin and urine protein concentrations

    c. Scr

    d. Neck vein distention at 30°

    e. Lymphangiogram

B. Before obtaining any of this information, you are told that a new chest x-ray shows pulmonary edema. Which **two** of the following diagnoses would be viable possibilities?

    a. Adverse effect of indomethacin

    b. Obstruction of the vena cava by tumor

    c. Renal failure

    d. Low albumin due to malnutrition

    e. Disuse of the muscles of the lower extremities

11. Which of the following is absolutely necessary to develop massive generalized edema?

    a. Renal Na^+ retention

    b. Blockage of lymphatic flow

    c. Increased intracapillary hydrostatic pressure

    d. Reduced intracapillary oncotic pressure

    e. Increased capillary wall permeability

chapter 3

Tonicity Disorders

Andrew S. Brem

The brain and kidneys function in tandem to regulate and maintain body water and solutes within narrow physiological boundaries. Chapter 1 summarizes how these two organ systems orchestrate such fine control over body fluid composition. Many commonly encountered diseases can directly or indirectly disrupt the homeostatic harmony of water and solute balance, resulting in either a hypertonic or hypotonic state in the affected patient. Diabetes insipidus, diabetes mellitus, severe diarrhea, heart failure, and tumors are but a few of the numerous clinical conditions which may perturb body fluid concentration. Since normal structure and function of the body cells require stable tonicity, failure of tonicity regulation can result in serious morbidity and mortality. This chapter will focus on some of the often seen disorders of body fluid tonicity, separating them into two broad categories—**hypertonic states** and **hypotonic states**—and will briefly cover the related problems of **polydipsia and polyuria.**

Physiologic Principles

Before discussing various clinical conditions, several basic physiologic principles should be mentioned for review purposes. **Osmolality** is a measure of the total number of particles dissolved in a kilogram of water. **Tonicity** assesses the solution's osmolar effect on water movement across semipermeable cell membranes. For example, if two solutions of unequal osmolality are separated by a semipermeable membrane, water will flow from the solution of low (hypotonic) to the solution of high osmolality (hypertonic). When the osmolality of both solutions becomes equal, isotonicity exists. Solutes such as urea which permeate cell membranes freely may increase total osmolality, but have no effect on tonicity as osmolality rises equally on both sides of all membranes and no water shifts occur. Since most cell membranes are freely permeable to water, one can assume that changes in tonicity within the extracellular space are matched by similar changes in the intracellular space.

The osmolality of the plasma mainly derives from Na^+ salts, urea and glucose. In fact, plasma osmolality can usually be assumed to be roughly equal to $2 \times$ serum Na^+ concentration, or can be estimated more precisely by the formula:

$$\text{Estimated osmolality} = 2[Na^+] + \frac{\text{BUN}}{2.8} + \frac{\text{glucose}}{18}$$

This estimate should approximate measured plasma osmolality within 10 mOsm/kg under normal conditions. If solute like ethanol unaccounted for by the formula is present in the plasma in substantial amounts or if the water content of the serum deviates from normal, the true measured osmolality can differ from this calculated value. Water and dissolved solutes like salts, urea and glucose normally make up 93% of serum volume with protein and lipid comprising the other 7%. Normal values of Na^+, BUN and glucose concentrations are based on the amount of these solutes present in a liter of plasma assuming a 93% aqueous phase. Increased protein or lipid concentration does not affect the osmolality of the aqueous phase, but decreases the percent volume of the aqueous phase of plasma, lowering measured Na^+, BUN and glucose.

Plasma osmolality mainly varies through addition or subtraction of water. As a rule, **change in plasma volume is related to change in Na^+ balance,** while **plasma osmolality correlates with water balance.** Under normal circumstances body osmolality is approximately 280–290 mOsm/kg despite wide fluctuations in dietary intake of solute and water. The kidney is the major organ responsible for this water and solute homeostasis.

If one assumes a normal metabolic rate and caloric intake, a 70-kg man generates approximately 600 mOsm of solute during a 24-hour period. Normally, the smallest urine volume in which the solute can be concentrated is approximately 500 ml with an osmolality of 1200 mOsm/kg. Conversely, the largest volume of urine in which this solute could be diluted is approximately 12 L with an osmolality of 50 mOsm/kg. Urine-specific gravity is a convenient bedside indicator of urine concentration and corresponds approximately to urine osmolalities as seen below:

Specific Gravity	Osmolality (mOsm/kg)
1.000	0
1.010	350
1.020	700
1.030	1050

Since plasma osmolality varies inversely with changes in total body water and blood volume may be independently affected by losses or gains in total body Na^+, one may encounter patients with abnormal plasma tonicity who are volume-contracted, euvolemic or volume-expanded. The following sections will consider these disorders of body tonicity and the related problem of polydipsia and polyuria.

Hypertonic States

Etiology

Hypertonicity is an increase in the effective osmolality of the body fluids to above the normal range. The osmotic effect of glucose in **hyperglycemia** (diabetes mellitus) may occasionally lead to a hypertonic state, but the osmotic effect of Na^+ in **hypernatremia** is by far the most common cause of hypertonicity. Hypernatremia is usually due to a deficit in body water, leading to an increase in the number of solute particles (Na^+) dissolved in a kilogram of water (Fig. 3.1). But rarely, an absolute increase in total body Na^+ without a loss of water leads to hypernatremia (e.g. administration of large amounts of concentrated $NaHCO_3$ during a cardiac arrest). The most important conditions producing hypertonic states are listed on Table 3.1.

DISEASE PROCESS

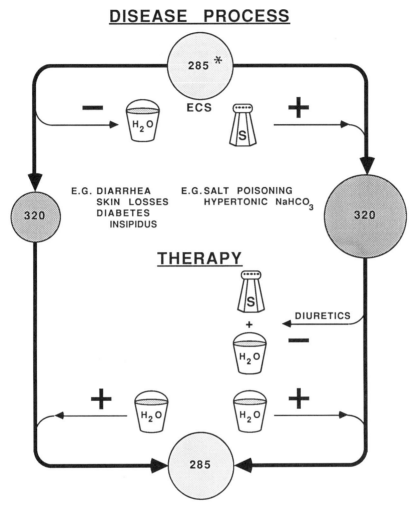

* OSMOLALITY (mOsm/kg)

Figure 3.1. Hypernatremia. Depiction of pathogenic mechanisms. **ECS** = extracellular space.

Table 3.1.
Principal Causes of Hypertonic States

I. Decreased water intake (increased serum Na^+ concentration)
  A. Inability to respond to thirst
    1. Inability to communicate
      a. Infants
      b. Altered sensorium
    2. Inability to swallow
    3. Lack of water source
  B. Defective thirst center
II. Water loss (increased serum Na^+ concentration)
  A. Extrarenal
    1. Diarrhea
    2. Vomiting
    3. Insensible loss
  B. Renal
    1. Central diabetes insipidus
      a. Hereditary
      b. Trauma
      c. Neoplasms
    2. Nephrogenic diabetes insipidus
      a. Hereditary
      b. Hypokalemia, hypercalcemia
      c. Pathological processes in the medulla
III. Solute gain
  A. Hyperglycemia (diabetes mellitus; reduced serum Na^+ concentration)
  B. Mannitol (reduced serum Na^+ concentration)
  C. Excessive intake of Na^+ (increased serum Na^+ concentration)
IV. Pseudohypertonicity: Increase in osmolality without change in tonicity
  A. Ingested substances
    1. Ethanol
    2. Methanol
    3. Ethylene glycol (antifreeze)
  B. High BUN

Pathogenesis

Water Deficit

Decreased Water Intake. The body's major defense against hypertonicity, be it from water loss or solute gain, is increased intake of water. An increase in plasma osmolality triggers the sensation of thirst, which then leads to an increased oral intake and correction of hypertonicity. Thus, hypertonicity usually develops in those unable to drink freely or to communicate thirst (typically young infants and aphasic or comatose individuals).

Increased Water Loss. Hypernatremia is most often produced by marked **extrarenal** losses of water in excess of Na^+. Examples include diarrheal dehydration in infants and small children and increased insensible losses from fever or high environmental temperature.

Hypernatremia can also result from excess **renal** water losses due to one of the forms of **diabetes insipidus (DI)**. **Central** DI results from a complete or partial failure of the posterior pituitary to secrete ADH. It can be due to inherited defects, trauma, neoplasms or other intracranial processes involving the supraoptic or paraventricular nuclei within the hypothalamus or the pituitary gland itself. Since patients may drink enough water to keep up with urinary losses and maintain normal tonicity, hypernatremia only occurs when an intercurrent illness interferes with water intake.

The obligate urinary water loss of DI may also be seen when the kidneys fail to respond to ADH. This failure to form a concentrated urine is referred to as **nephrogenic** DI. An inherited enzymatic defect may prevent the appropriate formation of 3′,5′-cyclic adenosine monophosphate (cAMP) in collecting duct epithelial cells after exposure to ADH. However, nephrogenic DI is more often an acquired and not an inherited disorder. Severe prolonged hypokalemia or hypercalcemia may result in a diminished renal response to ADH due, in part, to diminished generation of cAMP. Even when adequate cAMP is present, sickle cell disease, amyloidosis, chronic interstitial nephritis and urinary tract obstruction can all damage medullary structures, disrupting the normal medullary osmotic gradient necessary for ADH-induced water reabsorption. Thus, all of these conditions can lead to a urinary concentrating defect that is unresponsive to ADH.

Solute Gain

An increase in plasma osmolality can rarely occur with an absolute increase in body solute and not an excessive water loss. In clinical practice solutes such as glucose in diabetes mellitus and mannitol used in treating cerebral edema may achieve high concentrations in the extracellular fluid, where they produce hypertonicity. This results in passage of water from cells into the extracellular fluid leading to the dilution of other solutes, primarily Na^+. In these circumstances, hypertonicity is associated with hyponatremia! The expected dilution of extracellular Na^+ can be estimated in cases in which hyperglycemia exists; plasma Na^+ will be diluted by 1.6 mEq/L per 100 mg/dl increase in glucose concentration. Also, accidental feeding of formula with excessive NaCl to infants or use of concentrated $NaHCO_3$ has resulted in severe hypernatremia.

Pseudohypertonicity

The ingestion of ethylene glycol or alcohols such as methanol or ethanol may also increase measured plasma osmolality. However, tonicity is not changed, since these organic solutes pass freely into cells. They may cause a marked difference between the estimated and measured plasma osmolality.

Clinical Features

The main clinical effects of hypertonicity are neurologic signs, beginning with lethargy and confusion and progressing to seizures, coma and death. Central nervous system signs result from decreased brain volume as water moves out of brain cells into the hypertonic interstitial space.

Concomitant Na^+ loss may lead to signs and symptoms of volume depletion in situations such as diarrheal dehydration, or hyperglycemia with osmotic diuresis. Alternatively, the rare patients who received excessive administration of Na^+ may manifest hypervolemia.

High urine volumes (**polyuria**) will be seen in patients with DI and in those with hyperglycemia. Conscious patients will complain of thirst and may be drinking large amounts of fluid to keep up with the ongoing urinary losses (**polydipsia**).

Laboratory Features

High measured and calculated plasma osmolality is found in hypertonic states, but one may have elevated osmolality without hypertonicity when the solute is cell membrane permeable (e.g. ethanol, methanol, ethylene glycol and high BUN). Patients with hypertonicity due to mannitol or hyperglycemia often have hyponatremia but most other patients with increased body fluid tonicity demonstrate hypernatremia.

Diagnosis

Diabetics with hyperglycemic hypertonicity usually have normal or low serum Na^+ levels and are recognized by their blood or urine glucose levels.

Rare cases of hypernatremia due to excessive Na^+ intake can be recognized from a history of Na^+ administration and physical findings of hypervolemia. Other hypernatremic patients should be categorized according to their urine outputs and concentrations. Those with low volumes (~ 500 ml/day) and high concentrations (>600 mOsm/kg) usually have excessive extrarenal loss (diarrhea or high insensible losses). The other patients will have polyuria and a dilute urine caused by one of the forms of DI, which can be differentiated by the response to administration of ADH. A 50% rise in urine osmolality would be consistent with central DI and absence of response with nephrogenic DI.

Treatment

Hypertonicity is treated with intravenous administration of water as D5W or dilute saline solutions, depending on the concurrent need to administer Na^+. However, if the hypertonicity is complicated by hypovolemia, treatment initially should be directed toward correcting hypotension by replenishing the plasma volume deficit. Usually this is done with intravenous isotonic saline. After sufficient correction of volume to stabilize blood pressure and pulse, the water deficit should be gradually replaced as volume repletion continues. For example, most patients with hypernatremia secondary to diarrheal illness have lost Na^+ as well as water and therefore this water deficit replacement usually is with a dilute NaCl solution (0.2 normal saline in 5% dextrose).

If the hypernatremia is due to excessive intake of Na^+, it may be complicated by hypervolemia. This may be treated with diuretics, while the hypertonicity is treated with water replacement.

Hypernatremia should be corrected slowly in order to prevent brain swelling. During periods of hypertonicity, the brain cells generate osmotically active substances to partly balance the increase in extracellular osmolality. This generated intracellular solute reduces the shift of water out of the cell. If extracellular hypertonicity is corrected rapidly, the previously produced intracellular osmoles cause water to move into cells down an osmotic gradient and cell swelling results. Swelling of brain cells may cause an increase in intracranial pressure with lethargy, coma or seizures.

The amount of water that one needs to administer to correct hypernatremia may be calculated as shown in the example below:

An infant is admitted to hospital following a two-day history of diarrhea. Examination reveals a 10-kg lethargic infant with a pulse of 150/min and a blood pressure of 60/40 mm Hg. The serum Na^+ concentration is 170 mEq/L.

Estimated total body water in infants is 70% of body weight or 7 L. Estimated plasma osmolality is roughly 2 × serum Na^+ concentration or 340 mOsm/kg water. Therefore, total body osmoles are:

$$7 \text{ L} \times 340 \text{ mOsm/kg} = 2380 \text{ mOsm (sick state)}$$

Assume normal body osmoles = current body osmoles

$$285 \text{ mOsm/kg*} \times (\text{normal body water, L}) = 2380 \text{ mOsm}$$

*normal osmolality

$$\text{Normal body water (L)} = \frac{2380 \text{ mOsm}}{285 \text{ mOsm/kg}}$$

Normal body water (L) = 8.35 kg water or 8.35 L

Therefore, the water deficit = 8.35 L − 7 L or 1.35 L

Thus, 1.35 L must be given to this infant to correct the deficit. Once the hypotension is corrected with isotonic saline, replacement of the water deficit should occur over 36–48 hours. Ongoing losses should be added to the deficit replacement.

Treatment of underlying causes of hypertonicity should also be undertaken. In central diabetes insipidus, the ability to concentrate the urine can be restored by exogenous administration of ADH or by drugs such as chlorpropamide which may increase the renal responsiveness to suboptimal amounts of ADH. Nephrogenic diabetes insipidus has been treated with low sodium diets and low dose thiazide diuretics in an attempt to produce slight hypovolemia and increase proximal tubule reabsorption of salt and water. These patients continue to require free access to water. Hyperglycemia is treated with insulin.

Hypotonic States

Definition

Hypotonic states involve a decrease in the effective osmolality of the body fluids and result from a failure of the kidneys to excrete adequate amounts of free water. Hyponatremia is always an associated laboratory finding. Since hyponatremia can also be seen when the body's tonicity is high or normal, hypotonic ("true") hyponatremia should be distinguished from isotonic and hypertonic ("pseudo") hyponatremia.

Etiology

Table 3.2 lists the most important causes of hypotonicity. Patients often have more than one etiologic factor.

Table 3.2.
Principal Causes of Hypotonic States

I. Impaired water excretion (true hyponatremia)
  A. Volume depletion
    1. Whole blood loss-hemorrhage
    2. Plasma loss
      a. Renal (diuretics, aldosterone deficiency)
      b. Extrarenal (gastrointestinal loss, skin loss and third spacing)
  B. Euvolemic or slightly volume expanded states
    1. Tumors[a]
    2. Intracranial lesions[a]
    3. Lung diseases[a]
    4. Drugs[a]
    5. Thyroid and glucocorticoid deficiency
  C. Edematous states
    1. Renal failure
    2. Congestive heart failure
    3. Nephrotic syndrome
    4. Cirrhosis
II. Excess water intake, e.g. psychogenic polydipsia (true hyponatremia)
III. Pseudohypotonicity (pseudohyponatremia)
  A. Accumulation of non-Na^+ solutes (hypertonic hyponatremia)
    1. Glucose
    2. Mannitol
  B. Increased nonaqueous phase of plasma (isotonic hyponatremia)
    1. Hyperlipidemia
    2. Hyperproteinemia

---

[a]Syndrome of inappropriate ADH secretion.

Pathogenesis

Hypotonic states (true hyponatremia) usually come about through a renal defect in water excretion. This may be seen in patients with volume depletion, clinically normal volume or edematous states (Fig. 3.2). Rarely, excess water intake will result in hyponatremia despite normal renal water excretion.

Impaired Water Excretion

Volume Depletion. Hyponatremia may exist with volume depletion. This can be due to **extrarenal** losses from vomiting, diarrhea or third spacing. Alternatively, one may have excessive **renal** salt wasting from diuretics and aldosterone deficiency. One might think it unlikely for patients to become hypotonic in these situations because the fluids lost are usually more dilute than the plasma and initially body tonicity may rise. However, hypovolemia stimulates excessive thirst and the ensuing water intake not only corrects any early hypertonicity, but also can result in hyponatremia if renal water excretion is impaired.

The hypovolemic state stimulates ADH secretion and Na^+ reabsorption in the proximal tubule. The latter reduces delivery of tubular fluid to the diluting segment of the nephron (the ascending loop of Henle). Both this decreased distal delivery and increased ADH secretion prevent the kidney from excreting the water necessary to maintain water balance. Excess water accumulates, producing hyponatremia.

Euvolemia. Hyponatremia may exist when there is an absolute excess of total body water in the face of apparently **normal** extracellular volume. This form of hyponatremia results from an excess secretion of ADH in the absence of normal stimuli, such as hypovolemia or hypertonicity, and is called syndrome of inappropriate ADH secretion (SIADH). ADH may be produced from the pituitary gland directly or may be synthesized ectopically by various tumors. Patients have an inability to excrete free water reflected by an inappropriately concentrated urine in the presence of a low serum osmolality. Water retention produces subclinical hypervolemia. Thus, as the hyponatremia worsens and extracellular volume increases, the kidney may begin to waste Na^+, which prevents significant hypervolemia, but compounds the hyponatremia.

SIADH has a number of causes. As was mentioned, malignant tumors may produce ADH-like peptides. In addition, intracranial lesions such as brain abscess, tumor or meningitis, and pulmonary problems such as pneumonia, other lung diseases or ventilation with

DISEASE PROCESS

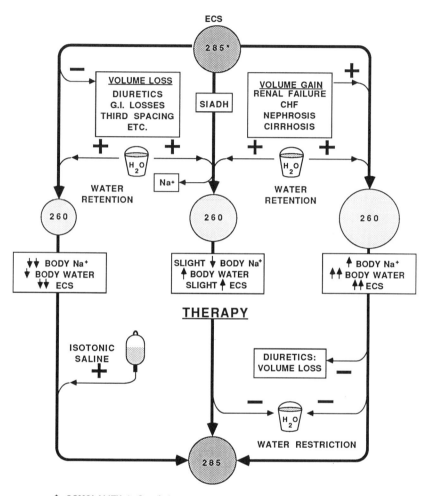

Figure 3.2. Hyponatremia due to impaired water excretion. Depiction of pathogenic mechanisms. **ECS** = extracellular space.

positive end expiratory pressure may stimulate the release of excess ADH. Pharmacologic agents also can produce SIADH. Examples include chlorpropamide, which enhances the renal response to ADH, and anesthetic agents and narcotics, which may stimulate the excessive release of ADH from the pituitary gland.

Hypothyroidism and glucocorticoid deficiency states also appear to be associated with an excessive release of ADH from the pituitary gland. The stimulus for this release is unclear.

Edematous States. Hyponatremia can exist when there is an excess extracellular volume, reflected by the presence of edema. The edematous states associated with hyponatremia include oliguric renal insufficiency, severe congestive heart failure, nephrotic syndrome and cirrhosis. In these examples, the hypotonic state results from limited excretion of ingested free water. Patients with oliguric renal failure are unable to produce large amounts of dilute urine because of a decrease in GFR. Patients with congestive heart failure, nephrotic syndrome or cirrhosis have decreased "effective" circulating volume which stimulates ADH secretion and reduces delivery of tubular fluid to the diluting segment of the nephron (the ascending limb of the loop of Henle). As a result, renal water excretion is impaired.

Excess Water Intake

This is a rare cause of hypotonicity since the patient's water intake must exceed the kidney's substantial capacity to excrete water, 10–20 L/day. Mentally ill individuals may manifest excessive drinking behavior called **psychogenic polydipsia** which can in extreme cases produce hypotonicity.

Clinical Features

The main clinical manifestations of hypotonic states are due to brain swelling and increased intracranial pressure as the brain cells take up water from the hypotonic extracellular space. Nausea and malaise may occur as the Na^+ concentration falls below 120 mEq/L. Headache and lethargy follow and seizures and coma are often seen with serum Na^+ levels below 110 mEq/L.

Patients may also show abnormal volume status and other clinical features of the primary condition that led to the hypotonicity.

Diagnosis

Hypotonic patients usually come to medical attention because of hyponatremia. The evaluation of hyponatremic patients begins with a plasma osmolality measurement to verify the hypotonicity, since there are two classes of conditions in which the finding of hyponatremia does not indicate the presence of hypotonicity.

Pseudohyponatremia

Hypertonic Hyponatremia. Hyponatremia may be due to the accumulation of non-Na^+ solutes in the extracellular fluid. As was mentioned in the discussion of pathogenesis of hypertonicity, glucose and mannitol may produce hyponatremia in the face of hypertonicity. A measurement of plasma osmolality will be high due to the presence of excess non-Na^+ osmoles.

Isotonic Hyponatremia. This is related to an increase in the non-aqueous phase of plasma. With severe **hyperlipidemia** or **hyperproteinemia** (in excess of 10 gm/dl), Na^+ concentration is reported as low; however, the measured osmolality will be normal and no real disturbances in body fluid tonicity are present.

True (Hypotonic) Hyponatremia

True hyponatremia is due to psychogenic polydipsia or a defect in renal water excretion. Although the history and physical examination usually allow one to distinguish these two categories of patients, the physician may confirm his impression with a urine osmolality, since the urine will be maximally dilute (Uosm <100 mOsm/kg; urine-specific gravity <1.003) in psychogenic polydipsia and less than maximally dilute in other cases.

It also may be instructive to collect a timed urine sample (typically an 8-, 12- or 24-hour collection) and calculate a free water clearance (C_{H2O}, may be expressed as ml/min or L/day).

$$C_{H2O} = V - C_{osm}$$

where V = urine volume, ml/min
C_{osm} = osmotic clearance, ml/min = $U_{osm}V/P_{osm}$
U_{osm} = urine osmolality, mosm/L
P_{osm} = plasma osmolality, mosm/L

Free water clearance mathematically defines the kidney's ability to conserve or excrete **solute-free water.** Free water clearance is positive when the urine is dilute and negative when the urine is concentrated. A patient with hyponatremia due to polydipsia should have maximum C_{H2O} (>8 L/day), while individuals with defective water excretion will have less than maximum C_{H2O} or even **negative C_{H2O}.** Sample calculation:

A 4-year-old boy is admitted to the hospital with meningitis. During his first 3 days of hospitalization his urine output decreases and he develops hyponatremia. Urine and plasma osmolalities are measured to determine free water clearance.

Plasma osmolality: 264 mOsm/kg

Urine osmolality: 310 mOsm/kg

Urine volume: 175 ml collected over 8 hours (0.36 ml/min)

$$C_{osm} = \frac{310 \text{ mOsm/kg } (0.36 \text{ ml/min})}{264 \text{ mOsm/kg}}$$

$$C_{osm} = 0.42 \text{ ml/min}$$

$$C_{H2O} = 0.36 \text{ ml/min} - 0.42 \text{ ml/min}$$

$$C_{H2O} = -0.06 \text{ ml/min or } - 86.4 \text{ ml/day}$$

Thus, rather than excreting free water to correct hyponatremia, 86.4 ml of free water/day are reabsorbed into the body accounting for the gradual development of hyponatremia.

Patients with true hypotonicity are classified according to their volume status on history and physical examination.

In the volume-depleted group, urine Na^+ concentration should be measured. Patients with extrarenal Na^+ losses usually conserve Na^+ appropriately in the urine and have urinary Na^+ concentrations of less than 20 mEq/L. On the other hand, urinary concentration of Na^+ is high, exceeding 30 mEq/L, in patients with renal Na^+ wasting and hyponatremia. Mineralocorticoid-deficient patients often demonstrate hyperkalemia in addition to the hyponatremia.

In patients with euvolemic hyponatremia, the kidneys waste Na^+ and urine Na^+ concentration usually is >30 mEq/L. Hypothyroidism and hypoadrenalism should be excluded by appropriate clinical or laboratory evaluation. Causes of SIADH will usually be apparent from the clinical picture.

Edematous patients are usually diagnosed by history, physical examination (e.g. signs of congestive heart failure) and routine tests, such as

BUN, Scr, serum albumin, urinalysis, chest X-ray and liver function tests.

Treatment

Specific therapy for the condition that causes hyponatremia obviously should be given, e.g. thyroxine for hypothyroidism. In the volume-depleted group treatment generally centers on replacement of the extracellular fluid deficit with normal saline. Correction of volume depletion will increase delivery of tubular fluid to the ascending loop of Henle and will allow the pituitary to respond appropriately to hypotonicity by turning off ADH secretion. Excess water will be excreted in the urine.

Most patients with SIADH or edematous states respond to restriction of free water intake. Excess body water is eliminated through insensible and urinary water loss. In addition, in edematous patients loop diuretics may be useful in controlling edema and may promote an increase in free water clearance by reversibly disrupting the medullary osmotic gradient.

At times the hyponatremia is severe enough to produce mental status changes. One may infuse hypertonic saline in order to raise serum Na^+ to 120–125 mEq/L and to rapidly reverse some of the central nervous system manifestations. Sample calculation:

A 50-kg woman with a known brain tumor is admitted to hospital confused and disoriented. Initial laboratory evaluation reveals a serum Na^+ concentration of 115 mEq/L and measured plasma osmolality of 230 mOsm/kg. How much 3% saline is needed to correct the serum Na^+ concentration to 125 mEq/L?

Assume total body water to be approximately 60% of weight or 30 L. Administer enough NaCl to raise osmolality of all body fluid spaces. Desired rise in serum Na^+: 125 − 115 mEq/L = 10 mEq/L

$$10 \text{ mEq/L} \times 30 \text{ L} = 300 \text{ mEq } Na^+ \text{ needed}$$

3% saline contains 0.52 mEq Na^+/ml (0.03 gm NaCl/ml × 1000 mg/gm × 1 mEq/58 mg NaCl)

$$300 \text{ mEq } Na^+ = X \text{ ml 3\% saline} \times 0.52 \text{ mEq } Na^+/\text{ml}$$

$$X = \sim 600 \text{ ml 3\% saline}$$

Polydipsia and Polyuria

Polydipsia or excessive thirst is an occasional problem seen by physicians. Patients typically drink large quantities of water and have large urine outputs (polyuria). This clinical picture can be caused by either form of **DI** or osmotic diuresis in **diabetes mellitus.** Despite the high urine volumes, these patients often are able to drink enough water to maintain *normal plasma Na$^+$ and osmolality levels.* Polydipsia and polyuria can also be seen in **psychogenic (primary) polydipsia.** Patients with psychogenic polydipsia usually have a very dilute urine and *normal plasma Na$^+$ and osmolality levels,* leading to confusion with patients with DI.

Patients with diabetes mellitus will be recognized by their hypertonic urine containing glucose. On the other hand, patients with psychogenic polydipsia and the two forms of DI have very dilute urine and can be differentiated by the **water deprivation test.** In this test the patient is weighed and then all fluids are restricted during the study period in order to deplete body water, increase tonicity and thereby stimulate ADH secretion. The test continues until either the patient loses 3% of his or her body weight or a concentrated urine is obtained. Generally, if 3% of the body weight is lost and the urine does not become concentrated, the patient is presumed to have some form of DI. At that point, ADH is administered to assess the renal response to exogenous hormone. A 50% rise in urine osmolality will be seen in central DI, while no response occurs in nephrogenic DI (Fig. 3.3).

Since patients with psychogenic polydipsia consume large quantities of free water chronically, they may wash out the medullary osmotic gradient present within the kidney. When they are water restricted in this test, at first many will fail to concentrate their urine maximally. In contrast to the clear response to ADH observed in central DI, ADH injection produces no further rise in urine osmolality. However, progressive water restriction will correct the concentrating defect.

Suggested Readings

DeFronzo RA and Thier SO. Pathophysiological approach to hyponatremia. Arch Int Med 1980;140:897–902.

Feig PU and McCurdy DK: The hypertonic state. NEJM 1977;297:1444–1454.

Gennari FJ: Serum osmolality, uses and limitations. NEJM 1984;310:102–105.

Goldman MB, Luchins DJ, and Robertson GL: Mechanisms of altered water

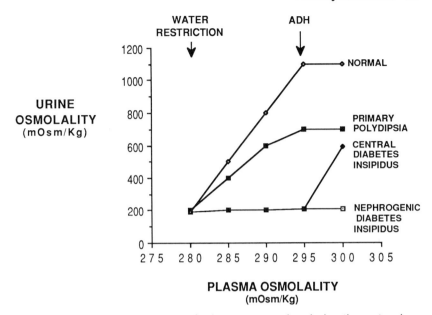

Figure 3.3. Typical responses of urine concentration during the water deprivation test. (Modified from Rose BD. Clinical physiology of acid-base and electrolyte disorders. 2nd ed. New York: McGraw-Hill Book Company, 1984:532.)

metabolism in psychotic patients with polydipsia and hyponatremia. NEJM 1988;318:397–403.

Katz MA: Hyperglycemia-induced hyponatremia. Calculation of expected serum Na$^+$ depression. NEJM 1973;289:843–844.

Rose BD: New approach to disturbances in the plasma sodium concentration. Am J Med 1986;81:1033–1040.

TONICITY DISORDER PROBLEMS

1. A 60-year-old man who was found unconscious in his apartment is brought to the emergency room by ambulance. A neighbor states that the patient has not felt well over the past week and looks as though he has lost weight lately. After an initial physical examination, laboratory studies are obtained. Match the data in Column A with the diagnosis in Column B.

Column A

	Serum Na$^+$ (mEq/L)	Plasma Osmolality (mOsm/kg)	Urine Osmolality (mOsm/kg)
1.	150	310	850
2.	150	310	200
3.	140	310	500
4.	125	310	500
5.	125	260	500

Column B
a. Diabetes mellitus (blood glucose concentration = 1000 mg/dl)
b. SIADH
c. Diabetes insipidus
d. Extra renal dehydration
e. Azotemia (BUN = 70 mg/dl)

2. A 22-year-old man with a brain tumor exhibits bizarre behavior and has a serum Na$^+$ concentration of 115 mEq/L. A 4-hour urine collection has a volume of 700 ml and an osmolality of 200 mOsm/kg. Midway during the collection a plasma osmolality of 250 mOsm/kg is obtained. Urine Na$^+$ concentration is 80 mEq/L.
   A. An appropriate urine osmolality with this plasma osmolality would be
      a. <100 mOsm/kg
      b. ~250 mOsm/kg
      c. >600 mOsm/kg
      d. Cannot tell from existing information
   B. An appropriate free water clearance in this setting would be
      a. Approximately −1 L/day
      b. Approximately +1 L/day
      c. >8 L/day
      d. Cannot tell from existing information
   C. Calculate the free water clearance
   D. The history and laboratory data suggest:
      a. SIADH
      b. Volume contraction secondary to third spacing
      c. Psychogenic polydipsia
      d. Volume contraction secondary to diarrhea
      e. Pseudohyponatremia
   E. What solution should be administered to the patient in question

2 to correct the serum Na^+ concentration to 120 mEq/L and how much would you give? Assume his weight to be 62 kg.

3. A. A 3-year-old boy presents to the hospital with edema for 3 days. Laboratory studies include a serum albumin of 1.5 gm/dl, a serum Na^+ 125 mEq/L, and heavy proteinuria is evident on a 24-hour urine collection. A laboratory technician also reports the serum as being very lipemic. The hyponatremia is likely due to:
   a. ADH
   b. Elevated blood lipids
   c. Either a or b
   d. Neither a nor b
   B. To clarify this question you could order a _____.

4. A patient with well-controlled insulin-dependent diabetes develops complete anuria because of obstruction. Then the patient omits a dose of insulin and serum glucose concentration rises rapidly. Would you expect the following parameters to rise, fall or remain unchanged due to the hyperglycemia?
   A. Plasma osmolality
   B. Plasma tonicity
   C. Serum Na^+ concentration
   D. Extracellular volume
   E. Intracellular volume

5. A known alcholic man is brought to the emergency room in a stupor. He was found by the police in a repair garage and several empty containers of antifreeze were nearby. On examination, he is tachypnic and is in a coma. A clever medical student orders serum chemistries and a plasma osmolality.

Na^+ 136 mEq/L	Cl^- 103 mEq/L	HCO_3^- 23 mEq/L
Glucose 80 mg/dl	Scr 1.2 mg/dl	K^+ 3.8 mg/L
BUN 30 mg/dl	Plasma osmolality 320 mOsm/kg	

   A. Calculate the expected plasma osmolality
   B. Is this patient in a hypotonic, hypertonic or isotonic state?
   C. The hyperosmotic state requires specific treatment with
      a. D5W
      b. ½ normal saline
      c. 3% saline
      d. General supportive care

6. An elderly woman is noted by her family to exhibit frequent urination. You perform a water deprivation test. Match the sets of laboratory data in column A with an appropriate diagnosis from column B.

Column A

		Urine Osmolality (mOsm/kg)	
Urine Volume/24 Hours	Baseline	H$_2$O Restriction	Post-ADH
1. 1000	610	905	900
2. 4000	187	188	820
3. 3500	201	198	203
4. 4000	102	623	631

Column B
a. Result of head trauma from an automobile accident
b. Chronic interstitial nephritis
c. Cystitis with frequent urination of small volumes
d. Alcoholic who is drinking 4–6 quarts of beer per day

7. A 2-year-old child weighing 22 lbs is admitted following a week of diarrhea and some vomiting. Serum Na$^+$ concentration is 160 mEq/L. Calculate the water deficit, assuming that the distribution of body fluid compartments is the same in an adult and baseline plasma osmolality is 285 mOsm/kg.

8. A 3-year-old child weighing 35 lbs is admitted to the hospital for surgical repair of bilateral partial urinary obstruction. Mother states: "He's always wet" and "He drinks a lot." In preparation for surgery scheduled the next day, he is given nothing by mouth after midnight. The next morning the surgical resident finds the child lethargic and febrile. Serum Na$^+$ concentration is 155 mEq/L and plasma osmolality is 315 mOsm/kg.
Two useful diagnostic tests would be:
a. A morning weight
b. Urine protein determination
c. Urine-specific gravity
d. Serum ethanol level
e. Water deprivation test

chapter 4

Acid-Base Disorders

David D. Clark

The physician frequently encounters acid-base disorders both in hospital and outpatient settings. Fortunately, these disorders are often mild and not central to clinical management, but at times an acid-base disorder is of critical importance in the care of a given patient. Therefore, it behooves the clinician to have a sound understanding of this complex and frequently misunderstood aspect of medicine.

Because free hydrogen ion (H^+) in solution is extraordinarily reactive, the body must regulate its concentration within narrow limits to allow for normal cellular and enzymatic function. Commonly, the concentration of H^+ is expressed in pH units. The normal pH value of extracellular fluid is 7.40 and the range of pH compatible with life is between 6.80 and 7.80.

Buffers

Buffering Mechanisms

All body fluids contain high concentrations of buffers that mainly consist of weak acids, HA, and their conjugate bases (or salts), A^-. These buffers in solution minimize changes in H^+ concentration when a strong acid or base is added to the solution.

For example:

Addition of acid: $\mathbf{H^+}$ $\mathbf{Cl^-}$ + Na^+ A^- $\rightleftharpoons$ Na^+ Cl^- + HA
strong   salt of   weak
acid   weak   acid
            acid

Addition of base: $\mathbf{Na^+}$ $\mathbf{OH^-}$ + HA $\rightleftharpoons$ Na^+ A^- + H_2O
strong
base

For a hypothetical weak acid, HA, and its conjugate base, A^-, the law of mass action is expressed as:

$$K_a = \frac{[H^+][A^-]}{[HA]} \qquad \text{equation 1}$$

where K_a is the dissociation constant for the buffer system. Rearranging,

$$[H]^+ = K_a \frac{[HA]}{[A^-]} \qquad \text{equation 2}$$

or, taking the negative logarithm,

$$pH = pK_a + \log \frac{[A^-]}{[HA]} \qquad \text{equation 3}$$

Thus, when $[A^-]/[HA] = 1$, the term $\log [A^-]/[HA] = 0$ and the pH of a given buffer system is equal to the pK_a of the system.

Optimum buffering, i.e. the ability to absorb added acid or base with minimum pH change, occurs in a pH range one unit above and below the pK_a of the buffer system. See the titration curve for the H_2CO_3/ HCO_3^- buffer system (Fig. 4.1).

The efficiency of any buffer pair will depend on two factors: concentration and pK_a. If two buffers have the same pK_a, the one with the greater concentration will buffer more H^+. If two buffers are present in the same concentration, the one whose pK_a is closest to the pH of the solution will be most efficient.

Extracellular fluid contains primarily HCO_3^- as a buffer and small amounts of phosphate and proteins. Intracellular fluid is buffered mainly by phosphate and proteins, including hemoglobin in red cells.

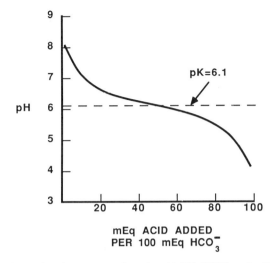

Figure 4.1. The titration curve for the H_2CO_3/HCO_3^- buffer system is shown. It can be seen that near the pK of 6.1 the pH changes little as acid is added to the system.

The H_2CO_3/HCO_3^- Buffer System

In chapter 1 we showed how the carbonic acid/bicarbonate (H_2CO_3/HCO_3^-) buffer pair can buffer either acid or base. In fact, this system plays a central role in acid-base homeostasis because: 1) ventilation can vary, thus controlling the partial pressure of CO_2(pCO_2) and in turn the concentration of H_2CO_3; and 2) renal excretion of acid can easily regenerate HCO_3^-, so that its concentration does not depend on intake. As a consequence, the H_2CO_3/HCO_3^- buffer pair deserves special consideration in the assessment of acid-base disorders.

The Henderson Equation

This is the law of mass action for the H_2CO_3/HCO_3^- buffer system. It expresses the relationship among pCO_2 and the concentrations of H^+ and HCO_3^- and is useful in the understanding of acid-base disorders.

The pCO_2, controlled by ventilatory function, determines the amount of CO_2 dissolved in body fluids. Cellular membranes are freely permeable to CO_2, so that extracellular pCO_2 is identical to intracellular pCO_2. In the presence of water and the ubiquitous enzyme, carbonic anhydrase, dissolved CO_2 equilibrates with H_2CO_3, which in turn equilibrates with HCO_3^- and H^+:

$$pCO_2 \rightleftharpoons \text{dissolved } CO_2 + H_2O \underset{\text{anhydrase}}{\overset{\text{carbonic}}{\rightleftharpoons}} H_2CO_3 \rightleftharpoons HCO_3^- + H^+$$

equation 4

This can be expressed, according to the law of mass action, as

$$\frac{[H^+]\,[HCO_3^-]}{[H_2CO_3]} = K_a;$$

equation 5

and, rearranging,

$$[H^+] = K_a \frac{[H_2CO_3]}{HCO_3^-]}$$

equation 6

Since H_2CO_3 is ultimately in equilibrium with pCO_2, it can be calculated by multiplying pCO_2 (expressed in mm Hg) by a constant, α.

$$[H^+] = K_a \frac{\alpha pCO_2}{[HCO_3^-]}$$

equation 7

Since K_a is a constant, and K_a times α is 24, this equation (the Henderson equation) can also be written

$$[H^+] = 24 \frac{pCO_2}{[HCO_3^-]}$$

equation 8

In human arterial plasma, the normal values are:

H^+ concentration = 40 nEq/L (range 38–43)
pCO_2 = 40 mm Hg (range 37–43)
HCO_3^- concentration = 24 mEq/L (range 22–28)

The Henderson-Hasselbalch Equation

Hasselbalch applied the concept of pH (negative logarithm of H^+ concentration) to the Henderson equation in order to facilitate the use of the more familiar pH units rather than H^+ concentration and thus "simplify" the Henderson equation. In fact, the original Henderson formulation is more convenient because deviations from normal values can be easily computed. Although pH can represent a wide range of H^+ concentration on a continuous scale from 0 to

14 and is thus useful in chemistry, its application to clinical medicine has probably only encumbered the assessment of acid-base disorders by requiring logarithmic calculations. Nevertheless, pH has become entrenched in clinical medicine.

The Hasselbalch variation of the Henderson equation is derived by taking the negative logarithm of the Henderson equation:

$$pH = pK_a + \log \frac{[HCO_3^-]}{[H_2CO_3]} \qquad \text{equation 9}$$

Likewise, equations 10 and 11 can be derived by taking the negative logarithm of equations 7 and 8, respectively.

$$pH = pK_a + \log \frac{[HCO_3^-]}{\alpha pCO_2} \qquad \text{equation 10}$$

$$pH = 6.1 + \log \frac{[HCO_3^-]}{0.0301\ pCO_2} \qquad \text{equation 11}$$

Whether one uses the Henderson or Henderson-Hasselbalch formulation, however, the important fact revealed by these equations is that it is not the absolute concentration of HCO_3^- or pCO_2, but rather the **ratio between the two** which reflects the H^+ concentration of a solution.

Overview of Acid-Base Disorders

Perturbations of H^+ homeostasis result from changes in HCO_3^- concentration or pCO_2.

Determinants of Bicarbonate Concentration

Rate of Hydrogen Ion Influx into the Extracellular Fluid

Metabolism of an average American diet produces 70–100 mEq of H^+ per day. The H^+ is a result of the metabolism of amino acid sulfhydryl groups to sulfuric acid and phospholipids to phosphoric acid, and the production of organic acids such as uric acid or creatinine. This "normal" generation of H^+ may be markedly increased in certain disease states such as lactic acidosis or ketoacidosis in which intermediary metabolism is disturbed and results in the accumulation of organic acids that are usually completely metabolized to CO_2 and H_2O (e.g. lactic acid, acetoacetic acid, etc.). With the increased production of H^+, HCO_3^- is consumed with the HCO_3^- concentration is reduced according to the reaction:

$$H^+ A^- + Na^+ HCO_3^- \rightleftharpoons H_2CO_3 + Na^+ A^- \qquad \text{equation 12}$$

Net Extrarenal Losses or Gains of Bicarbonate

Bicarbonate may be **lost** through diarrhea or drainage of alkaline pancreatic, biliary or small intestinal secretions via fistulae or tubes. Alternatively, HCO_3^- may be **gained** through a loss of HCl from vomiting or gastric drainage. The gastric loss of HCl is equivalent to an equimolar gain of $NaHCO_3$, since the gastric parietal cell produces HCl

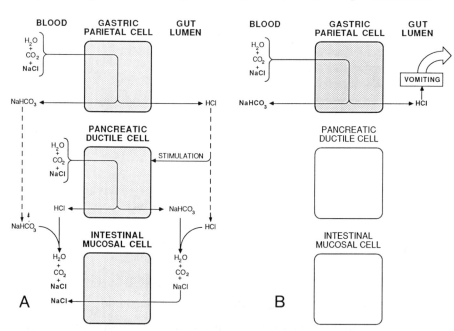

Figure 4.2. Diagram of HCO_3^- gain produced through gastric loss of HCl. (A) Normal: Stomach secretes HCl into the lumen and simultaneously generates $NaHCO_3$ in the blood. The pancreas neutralizes this process by secreting $NaHCO_3$ into the lumen and generating HCl in the blood. The NaCl formed in the lumen of the gut by the combination of $NaHCO_3$ and HCl is absorbed by the intestinal mucosal cells. (B) Vomiting: Loss of HCl from stomach reduces pancreatic production of $NaHCO_3$ and HCl. The $NaHCO_3$ generated by the stomach reenters the circulation and remains unneutralized.

from NaCl, H_2O and CO_2 and generates $NaHCO_3$ in the process (Fig. 4.2). Thus, when the HCl is lost through vomiting, the net result is a gain of $NaHCO_3$ and an increase in the HCO_3^- concentration along with a concomitant loss of Cl^- and a decline in the Cl^- concentration.

Net Renal Gains or Losses of Bicarbonate

Bicarbonate is (re)generated during the urinary excretion of acid (normally between 70 and 100 mEq/day) that is needed to balance the usual endogenous production of the same amount of H^+. In pathologic states excess acid excretion may lead to excess $NaHCO_3$ generation. HCO_3^- is **lost** through excretion of an alkaline urine.

Determinants of pCO_2 in Body Fluids

The rate of **CO_2 production** by cellular metabolism of tissues is relatively constant. Therefore, the rate of alveolar ventilation and **elimination of CO_2 by the lungs** ultimately determines the pCO_2 of body fluids, because alveolar ventilation can vary widely in response to a large number of physiologic and pathologic stimuli.

Definition of Primary Acid-Base Disorders

"Pure" Disorders

A **respiratory** acid-base disturbance is characterized by a primary change in pCO_2: **respiratory alkalosis** when pCO_2 is decreased and **respiratory acidosis** when pCO_2 is increased.

A **metabolic** acid-base disturbance is characterized by a primary change in HCO_3^- concentration: **metabolic acidosis** when HCO_3^- concentration is decreased and **metabolic alkalosis** when it is increased.

For example, in metabolic acidosis if HCO_3^- concentration is halved in the process of buffering a large H^+ load entering the extracellular fluid, the normal parameters would be changed as follows:

	pH	$[H^+]$	$K_a \cdot \alpha$	pCO_2	$[HCO_3^-]$	Henderson Equation
Normal	7.40	40	24	40	24	$40 = 24 \times \dfrac{40}{24}$
"Pure" metabolic acidosis:	**7.09**	**80**	24	40	**12**	$\mathbf{80} = 24 \times \dfrac{40}{\mathbf{12}}$

In the opposite case of a large HCO_3^- load entering the system, the doubling of $[HCO_3^-]$ would result in metabolic alkalosis

	pH	$[H^+]$	$K_a \cdot \alpha$	pCO_2	$[HCO_3^-]$	Henderson Equation
"Pure" metabolic alkalosis:	**7.70**	**20**	24	40	**48**	$20 = 24 \times \dfrac{40}{48}$

When pCO_2 is altered due to a change in ventilation, one develops respiratory alkalosis or acidosis:

	pH	$[H^+]$	$K_a \cdot \alpha$	pCO_2	$[HCO_3^-]$	Henderson Equation
"Pure" respiratory alkalosis:	**7.70**	**20**	24	**20**	24	$20 = 24 \times \dfrac{20}{24}$
"Pure" respiratory acidosis:	**7.09**	**80**	24	**80**	24	$80 = 24 \times \dfrac{80}{24}$

Actually the above "pure" conditions rarely occur in clinical practice.

Compensation

When a **primary metabolic** alteration occurs, it will be accompanied by a **secondary (compensatory) respiratory** change, which tends to diminish the change in H^+ concentration. Conversely, a **primary respiratory** alteration is accompanied by a **secondary (compensatory) metabolic** change.

In the following example of compensated metabolic acidosis, acidosis stimulates the brain respiratory center to increase ventilation and, hence, decrease pCO_2 which in turn moderates the change in $[H^+]$.

	ph	$[H^+]$	$K_a \cdot \alpha$	pCO_2	$[HCO_3^-]$	Henderson Equation
Normal:	7.40	40	24	40	24	$40 = 24 \times \dfrac{40}{24}$
"Pure" metabolic acidosis:	**7.09**	**80**	24	40	**12**	$80 = 24 \times \dfrac{40}{12}$
(Partially) "Compensated" metabolic acidosis:	**7.30**	**50**	24	**25**	12	$50 = 24 \times \dfrac{25}{12}$

In the next example of compensated respiratory acidosis, plasma HCO_3^- concentration has increased as a result of both buffering and increased renal H^+ excretion (see section on **respiratory acidosis**).

pH $[H^+]$ $K_a \cdot \alpha$ pCO_2 $[HCO_3^-]$ Henderson Equation

Normal:	7.40 40	24	20	24	$40 = 24 \times \dfrac{40}{24}$
"Pure" respiratory acidosis:	**7.09 80**	24	**80**	24	$80 = 24 \times \dfrac{80}{24}$
(Partially) "Compensated" respiratory acidosis:	**7.22 60**	24	80	**32**	$60 = 24 \times \dfrac{80}{32}$

It should be noted that respiratory compensation of either metabolic acidosis or alkalosis is more rapid and effective than metabolic compensation of primary respiratory alterations. Also, compensation for the primary alteration will not be sufficient to restore a normal H^+ concentration, and consequently the **compensation will be only partial.**

Complex Acid-Base Disorders

Rarely, two opposing primary processes may exist at the same time. For example, a patient with primary respiratory alkalosis with metabolic compensation may have the following picture:

pH $[H^+]$ $K_a \cdot \alpha$ pCO_2 $[HCO_3^-]$ Henderson Equation

7.51   32   24   24   18 $32 = 24 \times \dfrac{24}{18}$

If this patient then develops a second disorder resulting in HCO_3^- losses (superimposed primary metabolic acidosis), the net results would be a pattern of primary respiratory alkalosis **and** superimposed primary metabolic acidosis, as follows:

pH $[H^+]$ **72** $K_a \cdot \alpha$ pCO_2 $[HCO_3^-]$ Henderson Equation

7.15   24   24   8 $72 = 24 \times \dfrac{24}{8}$

Since the final H^+ concentration may be higher than normal despite the respiratory alkalosis, the term **acidemia** is used to denote the presence of a higher than normal H^+ concentration. In the example given above, the alteration in H^+ metabolism could be described as: Respiratory alkalosis with superimposed metabolic acidosis resulting in acidemia. In other situations the term **alkalemia** may apply.

Metabolic Acidosis

As previously defined, metabolic acidosis results from any disorder which causes a **primary reduction in plasma HCO_3^- concentration.** A plasma HCO_3^- concentration less than 15 mEq/L is almost always due to metabolic acidosis rather than compensation for respiratory alkalosis (see section on **respiratory alkalosis**).

This condition is common, and when severe is a medical emergency. Death may be caused either by the underlying process responsible for the acidosis, or by the acidosis itself, or occasionally by the accompanying hyperkalemia (to be discussed in the chapter on **potassium disorders**).

Etiology

Some common and important causes of metabolic acidosis are listed in Table 4.1.

Pathophysiology

General Comments

Metabolic acidosis occurs whenever the influx of H^+ into the extracellular fluid is more rapid than the capacity of the kidney to excrete the H^+ into the urine. This influx may occur through two basic mechanisms a) **endogenously produced acid** (e.g. ketoacidosis) or b) **loss of HCO_3^-** (e.g. diarrhea). Also, exogenously administered acid, e.g. HCl, is another mechanism; it is rare and will not be discussed further.

Integrated Response to an Acid Load

We will examine the integrated response of the organism when a large H^+ load is presented to the extracellular fluid (Fig. 4.3).

Buffering. Pitts has shown that about 43% of an H^+ load administered as HCl is buffered extracellularly: 42% by titration of HCO_3^- (H^+ + HCO_3^- → H_2CO_3 → H_2O + CO_2) and 1% by proteins (H^+ + Pr^- → HPr). The remaining 57% is buffered intracellularly, mainly by

Table 4.1.
Principal Causes of Metabolic Acidosis

I. Increased Anion Gap
  A. Ketoacidosis
    1. Diabetes mellitus
    2. Starvation
  B. Lactic acidosis
  C. Ingestions
    1. Salicylates
    2. Methyl alcohol
    3. Ethylene glycol
  D. Renal failure
II. Normal Anion Gap
  A. Loss of alkaline intestinal secretions (hypokalemic)
    1. Diarrhca
    2. Fistulae
    3. Biliary or pancreatic drainage tubes
  B. Acetazolamide (hypokalemic)
  C. Renal tubular acidosis (hypokalemic)
    1. Proximal
    2. Distal
  D. Aldosterone deficiency (hyperkalemic)
    1. Primary adrenal insufficiency
    2. Hyporeninemic hypoaldosteronism
    3. Inhibitors of aldosterone effect (K^+ sparing diuretics)
      a. Spironolactone
      b. Triamterene
      c. Amiloride

phosphate and proteins. Most H^+ enters cells in exchange for Na^+ and K^+, which are released from intracellular buffers during titration by H^+.

Examples:

$$1) \text{ Na proteinate} + H^+ \rightarrow \text{H protein} + Na^+ \quad \text{equation 13}$$

$$2) \text{ Na}_2\text{HPO}_4 + H^+ \rightarrow \text{NaH}_2\text{PO}_4 + Na^+ \quad \text{equation 14}$$

This first line of defense minimizes changes in H^+ concentration but is accompanied by a persistent increase in the total H^+ present in the organism.

Respiratory Compensation. Secondly, as a result of increased cerebral H^+ concentration, the respiratory center is stimulated and ventilation increases, reducing pCO_2. The ratio of H_2CO_3 to HCO_3^- falls

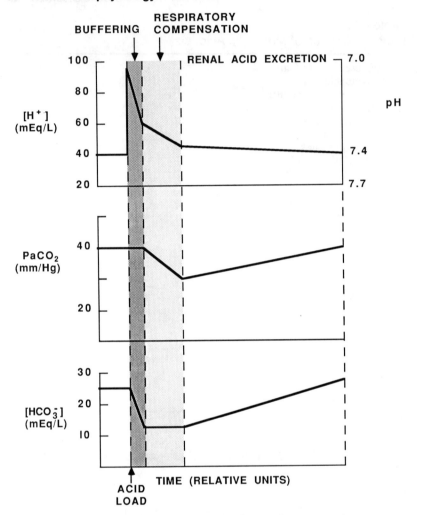

Figure 4.3. Schematic representation of the three phases of defense against an acid load: buffering, respiratory compensation and definitive correction (renal acid excretion).

toward normal, but does not, however, correct completely. Therefore, **H^+ concentration will approach, but not quite reach, normal.**

Definitive Correction. Thirdly, renal net acid excretion will increase mainly via an increase in excretion of ammonium. Over a period of hours to days, depending on the level of renal function and the size and duration of the H^+ load, all H^+ which entered the system will be eliminated and the amount of H^+ in the organism will be restored to normal. Although buffering and respiratory compensation help prevent large changes in H^+ concentration, **only the elimination of the H^+ load by the kidney is capable of restoring acid-base homeostasis.** (The mechanism of renal acid excretion was covered in the chapter on **review of normal physiology.**)

Increased Anion Gap

In order to maintain electroneutrality, the sum of all cations in body fluids must equal the sum of all anions. The cations in extracellular fluid are normally made up of Na^+ ($\sim$140 mEq/L), K^+ ($\sim$4.5 mEq/L), Ca^{2+} ($\sim$5 mEq/L) and small concentrations of Mg^{2+} and other substances. The anions are Cl^- ($\sim$105 mmEq/L), HCO_3^- ($\sim$24 mEq/L), proteins ($\sim$15 mEq/L), as well as phosphate, sulphate, amino acids, urate, lactate, etc. In practice only Na^+, K^+, Cl^- and HCO_3^- are measured as part of the "electrolyte" profile. Thus an equivalence between the total cations and anions in blood can be expressed:

$[Na^+]$ + $[K^+]$ + [unmeasured cations]
$\qquad$ = $[Cl^-]$ + $[HCO_3^-]$ + [unmeasured anions]$\qquad$ equation 15

The anion gap is defined and calculated as the term $[Na^+]$ − ($[Cl^-]$ + $[HCO_3^-]$) and is thus equivalent to the [unmeasured anions] − ([unmeasured cations] + $[K^+]$) (equation 15 rearranged). Since gross changes in the concentration of unmeasured cations and K^+ do not occur except in unusual circumstances, **changes in the anion gap are determined primarily by the unmeasured anions.** The normal anion gap, calculated as $[Na^+]$ − ($[Cl^-]$ + $[HCO_3^-]$), is 8–14 mEq/L.

With metabolic acidosis due to addition of acid, the fundamental reaction of buffering by HCO_3^- is:

$$H^+A^- + Na^+\,HCO_3^- \rightleftharpoons H_2CO_3 + Na^+A^- \qquad \text{equation 16}$$

As acid is added, HCO_3^- will "disappear" as it is converted to H_2CO_3 (which is in equilibrium with dissolved CO_2 and H_2O, see above). The acid anion, A^-, will "appear" in plasma instead of the HCO_3^-. If the acid is HCl, then as the HCO_3^- concentration decreases, the Cl^- concentration will increase reciprocally. The calculated anion gap will not change as both HCO_3^- concentration and Cl^- concentration are measured and the term $([HCO_3^-] + [Cl^-])$ will not change. If, on the other hand, the acid anion, A^-, is not routinely measured (e.g. lactic acid), then the HCO_3^- concentration will decrease but there will be no reciprocal increase in Cl^- concentration and the term $([HCO_3^-] + [Cl^-])$ will decrease, resulting in an increase in the calculated anion gap. Stated alternatively, the concentration of the unmeasured acid anion, A^-, in plasma will have increased.

With metabolic acidosis due to loss of HCO_3^-, Cl^- retention reciprocally increases Cl^- concentration for the decrease in HCO_3^- concentration. Hence, the calculated anion gap will not be changed. In HCO_3^- loss from diarrhea the reciprocal gain in Cl^- occurs because the gastrointestinal tract cells that secrete HCO_3^- simultaneously produce HCl (Fig. 4.4). If the $NaHCO_3$ is not reabsorbed by the gut, the overall result is the generation of HCl. In HCO_3^- loss in the urine, increased renal Na^+ avidity increases Na^+ reabsorption with Cl^-, the only other anion available to the kidney for reabsorption with Na^+.

Specific Disorders Causing Anion Gap Acidosis

The principal causes of anion gap acidosis are conditions that add organic or other acids to the body faster than the kidneys can excrete them.

Ketoacidosis. This is mainly seen in fasting and diabetes mellitus. It is brought about by low insulin and high glucagon levels. Lipolysis in

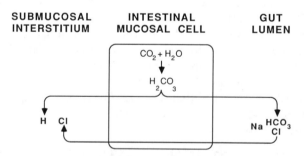

Figure 4.4. Production of HCl by intestinal mucosal cells in patients with diarrhea. A HCO_3^-/Cl^- exchanger at the luminal surface converts NaCl in the gut lumen to $NaHCO_3$. In the process, HCl is secreted into the submucosal interstitium and absorbed into the blood.

adipose tissue increases production of fatty acids which are converted in the liver to the ketoacids, β-hydroxybutyric and acetoacetic acid. In diabetes mellitus insulin deficiency also produces hyperglycemia.

Lactic Acidosis. This is due to accumulation of lactic acid. It may be seen in a variety of conditions, but occurs mainly in states of decreased tissue perfusion. The lack of oxygen impairs conversion of NADH to NAD^+ and metabolism of pyruvate by the Krebs cycle. The high levels of NADH promote conversion of pyruvic to lactic acid which regenerates NAD^+ needed for glycolysis, but may rapidly lead to severe, life-threatening acidosis.

Salicylate Ingestion. This is characterized by varying combinations of two primary acid-base disorders: respiratory alkalosis due to salicylate-induced stimulation of the respiratory center and metabolic acidosis due to accumulation of unknown acids (?lactic, ?salicylic, ?other).

Methyl Alcohol or Ethylene Glycol Ingestion. Acidosis is due to formation of metabolites of these compounds (formic acid for methyl alcohol, oxalic acid for ethylene glycol), as well as to increased formation of lactic acid and possibly other organic acids.

Renal Failure. In this instance, the acidosis is due to the decreased ability of the kidney to excrete a normal H^+ load. The anion gap is increased by phosphate, sulfate and other anions that accumulate due to the reduced GFR. These two processes parallel one another and, hence, a metabolic acidosis with an elevated anion gap ensues.

Specific Disorders Causing Normal Anion Gap Acidosis

The principal causes of metabolic acidosis with a normal anion gap are intestinal or renal HCO_3^- losses and renal excretion of less acid than the amount produced from the diet.

Loss of Alkaline Intestinal Secretions. This is seen most commonly with diarrhea or drainage of other alkaline intestinal fluids. These secretions contain significant amounts of HCO_3^- and, in the case of diarrhea, K^+.

Administration of Acetazolamide. This agent inhibits carbonic anhydrase and blocks HCO_3^- reabsorption by the proximal tubule, resulting in HCO_3^- (and Na^+) diuresis.

Renal Tubular Acidosis (RTA). Acidosis may be caused by inability of the distal tubule to maximally lower urine pH ("distal" RTA) or by a defect in the proximal tubule's reabsorption of HCO_3^- ("proximal" RTA). In either case, there is inadequate renal H^+ secretion resulting in either impaired renal HCO_3^- reabsorption ("proximal RTA") or impaired renal HCO_3^- regeneration ("distal RTA"). Thus, the kidneys cannot maintain acid-base homeostasis. RTA occurs with a normal or near normal GFR, and is, therefore, not associated with an increased anion gap as in renal failure. Either type may be inherited or acquired. Either type may occur as a primary transport defect or as a complication of an interstitial or tubular disorder such as pyelonephritis. The proximal variety can also be associated with other disorders of the proximal tubule involving defective reabsorption of phosphate, glucose, amino acids and urate (Fanconi's syndrome). The distal variety is associated with hypercalciuria and nephrocalcinosis. Hypokalemia due to renal K^+ wasting is seen in both types of RTA.

Aldosterone Deficiency. This leads to decreased Na^+-H^+ and Na^+-K^+ "exchange" in the cortical collecting tubule. Reduced excretion of K^+ and H^+ and impaired renal HCO_3^- regeneration result in **hyperkalemia** and acidosis. This may be due to adrenal gland failure, an isolated aldosterone deficiency or drugs which block aldosterone effect (spironolactone, triamterene, amiloride).

Clinical Features

The clinical manifestations of metabolic acidosis are usually those of the underlying disorder; however, with severe acidosis, patients can present with Kussmaul's respirations (deep respirations due to severe hyperventilation), hypotension, cardiac arrhythmias, and changes in level of alertness progressing to coma. Severe acidemia (pH <7.00 to 7.15) results in impaired cardiac contractility, massive release of endogenous catecholamines predisposing to cardiac arrhythmias and peripheral vasodilation. These latter factors probably explain the hypotension (frequently unresponsive to vasopressors) seen with severe metabolic acidosis.

Treatment

Ideally, one should reverse the causative process. For example, this can be done with insulin in diabetes mellitus or by stopping drugs that block aldosterone. When this is not possible, or when the acidosis is severe and life-threatening (pH $\leq$7.15; HCO_3^- $\leq$8 mEq/L), $NaHCO_3$ should be given in amounts adequate to correct the acidosis at last **partially** (pH $\geq$7.20; HCO_3^- $\geq$10 mEq/L). In this situation one may calculate the dose of $NaHCO_3$ by multiplying the desired change in plasma HCO_3^- concentration by 50% of the body weight in kilograms. For example, a 70-kg man with a HCO_3^- concentration of 5 mEq/L would require 35 L $\times$ 5 mEq/L or 175 mEq $NaHCO_3$ to raise his serum HCO_3^- concentration to 10 mEq/L.

When the acidosis is due to accumulation of acid anions that can be metabolized (acetoacetate, lactate, etc.), reversal of the underlying process may lead to "regeneration" of HCO_3^-

$$CH_3\,CHOH\,COO^-\,Na^+ + 3O_2 \rightarrow 2\,CO_2 + 2\,H_2O + NaHCO_3$$
$(Na^+$ lactate) $\hspace{4cm}$ equation 17

and spontaneous correction of the acidosis. In this case, if large amounts of HCO_3^- had previously been administered, the "conversion" of the organic anion back to HCO_3^- could cause metabolic alkalosis ("overshoot alkalosis").

Occasionally, K^+ disturbances are the most immediately dangerous consequences of metabolic acidosis. Diarrhea and RTA are associated with K^+ losses in the stool and urine, respectively. Osmotic induced urinary K^+ losses also occur in diabetic acidosis (see chapter on **potassium disorders**). Correction of the acidosis promotes the reentry of K^+ into cells. If serum K^+ concentration is normal or low in acidosis, correction of the acidosis may result in severe hypokalemia. K^+ administration is necessary in these instances. Hyperkalemia due to metabolic acidosis will be discussed in the chapter on **potassium disorders.**

In addition to these considerations, attention should be paid to the degree of respiratory compensation. A "rule of thumb" may be useful in detecting whether the respiratory compensation is adequate: in chronic metabolic acidosis pCO_2 decreases by about 1.2 $\pm$ 0.3 mm Hg for each milliequivalent per liter of decrease in HCO_3^- concentration from normal. Thus, with a HCO_3^- concentration of 14 mEq/ L, one might expect a pCO_2 of about 28 mm Hg and a H^+ concentration of 48 nEq/L, for a pH of 7.32. Respiratory compensation to acute metabolic acidosis is even more pronounced. If pCO_2 fails to decrease appropriately, the patient may be suffering from pulmonary disease and the degree of acidosis will be more severe than that usually seen for the same value of HCO_3^- concentration in a patient with normal respiratory compensation. Therapy should therefore be directed not only at correcting the metabolic acidosis, but also toward the respiratory system.

Metabolic Alkalosis

As defined above, metabolic alkalosis results from any disorder that causes a **primary increase in plasma HCO_3^- concentration.** A plasma HCO_3^- concentration greater than 35 mEq/L is almost always due to metabolic alkalosis rather than compensation for respiratory acidosis (see section on **respiratory acidosis**).

Etiology

Table 4.2 lists the main causes of metabolic alkalosis, the most common of which are diuretics and vomiting.

Table 4.2.
Principal Causes of Metabolic Alkalosis

I. Loss of acid (urine Cl^- <15 mEq/L)
   A. Extrarenal
      1. Vomiting
      2. Gastric drainage
   B. Renal
      1. Diuretics[a]
         a. Thiazides
         b. Furosemide
         c. Ethacrynic acid
      2. Posthypercapneic alkalosis
II. Gain of Alkali (urine Cl^- >20mEq/L)
   A. Rapid administration of $NaHCO_3$
   B. Primary mineralocorticoid excess
      1. Endogenous
         a. Primary aldosteronism
         b. Cushing's disease
      2. Exogenous
         a. High dose corticosteroid administration
         b. Disorders simulating mineralocorticoid excess[b]
            i. Licorice
            ii. Chewing tobacco
      3. Primary aldosteronism

---

[a]If the diuretic agent has been given recently, urine Cl^- may be > 15 mEq/L, as a result of the direct chloriuretic action.
[b]Licorice acts with a mechanism similar to that of corticosteroids because of the properties of its basic constituent, glycyrrhizic acid. Chewing tobacco also contains glycyrrhizic acid.

Pathophysiology

Production of Metabolic Alkalosis

A primary increase in plasma HCO_3^- concentration can be **produced** through a **loss of acid** or **gain of alkali**. These are the mirror images of the processes that cause metabolic acidosis and will be discussed in more detail under the specific causes of metabolic alkalosis.

Maintenance of Alkalosis

Unlike metabolic acidosis, however, the **maintenance** of a persistently elevated plasma HCO_3^- concentration requires a failure of renal HCO_3^- excretion. When there has been an increase in plasma HCO_3^- concentration, the kidney is ordinarily capable of excreting the excess HCO_3^-. Since the total extracellular HCO_3^- is filtered by the kidney more than 10 times/day (HCO_3^- filtered per day = 140 L glomerular filtrate/day $\times$ 24 mEq HCO_3^-/L = 3360 mEq HCO_3^-/day), a small difference between HCO_3^- filtration and reabsorption may greatly alter HCO_3^- excretion. For example, if the tubule permits just 2% of the filtered HCO_3^- to be excreted, about 70 mEq/day will be lost in the urine, thus lowering plasma HCO_3^- concentration and correcting metabolic alkalosis. The failure of this regulating mechanism to occur in ongoing metabolic alkalosis is due to increased tubular $NaHCO_3$ reabsorption.[a]

The overall level of tubular $NaHCO_3$ reabsorption can be modulated not only by extracellular pH, but also by a variety of other factors. Alterations which tend to increase tubular $NaHCO_3$ reabsorption are listed on Table 4.3. In the maintenance of most types of metabolic alkalosis, increased aldosterone level, increased tubular Na^+ reabsorption and decreased availability of Cl^- for reabsorption with Na^+ are the most important determinants. Let us examine in some detail what happens to tubular $NaHCO_3$ reabsorption when plasma HCO_3^- concentration increases as a result of a) loss of H^+ through vomiting or b) administration of HCO_3^-.

During vomiting, the loss of H^+ and Cl^- from the stomach increases plasma HCO_3^- concentration (Fig. 4.2), i.e. produces alkalosis and reduces plasma Cl^- concentration. As a result, the glomerular filtrate contains more HCO_3^- and less Cl^-. Concurrently, the loss of water and

---

[a]Tubular $NaHCO_3$ reabsorption occurs through the combination of H^+ secretion, Na^+ reabsorption and HCO_3^- generation that was covered in the chapter on **review of normal physiology**.

Table 4.3.
Factors That Increase Tubular Bicarbonate Reabsorption

Increased	Decreased
Plasma aldosterone concentration Tubular Na^+ reabsorption pCO_2	Tubular fluid Cl^- available for reabsorption with Na^+ Body K^+ pH

small amounts of Na^+ and K^+ in the vomitus result in volume depletion, increased renal Na^+ retention and increased release of aldosterone. In the face of the increased aldosterone level and tubular Na^+
reabsorption and reduced Cl^- available for reabsorption with Na^+, an
increase in tubular $NaHCO_3$ reabsorption prevents excretion of the
increased filtered HCO_3^- and the elevated plasma HCO_3^- concentration persists. Due to decreased filtered Cl^- and increased tubular reabsorption of Cl^- along with Na^+, **the urine is virtually Cl^--free.** In addition, high aldosterone levels increase renal K^+ and H^+ secretion, thus
resulting in urinary K^+ losses, hypokalemia and often an acid urine.
(Acid urine in the face of alkalemia has been called paradoxical
aciduria).

This contrasts with the response to the administration of $NaHCO_3$.
Plasma HCO_3^- concentration increases along with body Na^+ stores
and extracellular volume. The aldosterone level and tubular Na^+ reabsorption are both reduced and there is adequate Cl^- available for reabsorption with Na^+ at this low rate of tubular Na^+ reabsorption. As a
result of this decreased aldosterone level and renal Na^+ reabsorption
along with the availability of Cl^- for reabsorption with Na^+, tubular
$NaHCO_3$ reabsorption decreases, resulting in excretion of the excess
$NaHCO_3$ and return of body Na^+ stores and plasma HCO_3^- concentration to normal. Thus, alkalemia in this situation is brief.

Integrated Response to a Base Load

As outlined above for metabolic acidosis, the integrated response to
metabolic alkalosis consists of first **buffering,** second **respiratory compensation** and third **definitive correction,** which occurs via a change in
renal function.

Buffering. In metabolic alkalosis about one-third of an administered HCO_3^- load is titrated by the movement of H^+ out of cells and two-thirds remains in the extracellular space, thus increasing the plasma HCO_3^- concentration.

Respiratory Compensation. Compensation for metabolic alkalosis consists of decreased ventilation which results in an increased pCO_2.[b] The response is incomplete because decreased alveolar ventilation induced by the change in pH causes some degree of hypoxemia which in turn is a stimulus to ventilation. The net result of the hypercapnia is to return the ratio of H_2CO_3 to HCO_3^- toward normal; hence, the **H^+ concentration and pH approach, but do not reach normal values.**

Definitive Correction. This requires a change in renal function resulting in **reduced tubular $NaHCO_3$ reabsorption.** Thus, the kidneys excrete the excess HCO_3^- and correct the metabolic alkalosis.

Specific Disorders Producing Metabolic Alkalosis

As mentioned above, metabolic alkalosis can be **produced** by loss of acid or gain of alkali.

Metabolic Alkalosis due to Acid Losses. The majority of patients with persistent metabolic alkalosis are in this category. The acid lost is HCl; it can be lost **through the gastrointestinal tract** through vomiting or gastric drainage (Fig.4.5B), or **through the kidney** as occurs following most diuretics (Fig. 4.6B), or in posthypercapneic metabolic alkalosis.

In the case of **diuretic administration** urinary NaCl losses lead to a decrease in effective circulating volume, which in turn stimulates aldosterone secretion and tubular Na^+ reabsorption. This enhances renal tubular $NaHCO_3$ generation, adding $NaHCO_3$ to the blood and converting NaCl in the urine to HCl (actually NH_4Cl) which is excreted.

Due to the Cl^- depletion induced by the diuretics, patients chronically on diuretics and a low-salt diet will have **low urine Cl^-. However, Cl^- may appear transiently in the urine** after the patient takes each dose.

Posthypercapneic metabolic alkalosis occurs in hypovolemic patients who are recovering from respiratory failure.

---

[b]The degree of increase in pCO_2 is roughly 0.7 mm Hg (range 0.5–1.0 mm Hg) for every mEq/L increase in HCO_3^- concentration above normal. However, it is uncommon for the pCO_2 to rise above 55 mm Hg.

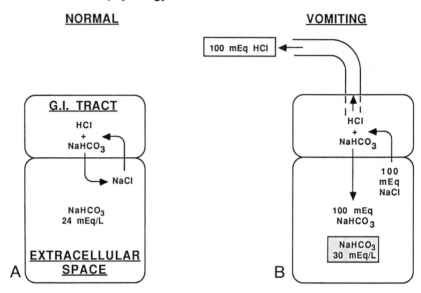

Figure 4.5.   Production of metabolic alkalosis from vomiting. (A) Normal. Luminal HCl produced in the stomach combines with luminal $NaHCO_3^-$ produced in the pancreas and is reabsorbed into the extracellular fluid. (B) Gastric loss of HCL. Loss of 100 mEq would leave 100 mEq $NaHCO_3$ behind in body.

With hypercapnia renal losses of HCl occur as compensation for respiratory acidosis and lead to a compensatory increase in plasma HCO_3^- concentration. Sodium and Cl^- depletion and enhanced aldosterone secretion are coincidentally produced by a low salt diet or diuretics. Metabolic alkalosis develops when the patient's pCO_2 is returned toward normal. In the absence of adequate administration of Cl^- and the presence of high aldosterone levels and tubular Na^+ reabsorption, increased tubular $NaHCO_3$ reabsorption maintains the alkalosis. Again **urine Cl^- will be low.**

Metabolic Alkalosis due to Gain of Alkali. The **administration of $NaHCO_3$** is not accompanied by persistent alkalosis unless the rate of administration is rapid (see section on **maintenance of alkalosis**).

Clinically, the conditions which most often result in metabolic alkalosis through gain of alkali are those associated with **excessive mineralocorticoid activity,** which increases Na^+ reabsorption, new HCO_3^-

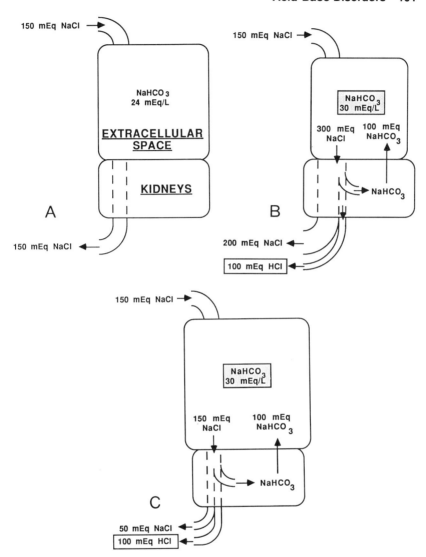

Figure 4.6   (A) Normal. Daily urinary NaCl excretion balances ingestion. (B) Diuretics result in excessive urinary NaCl loss, extracellular volume depletion and conversion of extracellular NaCl to $NaHCO_3$. (C) Mineralocorticoid excess. NaCl that should be excreted is converted to HCl that is eliminated in the urine and $NaHCO_3$ that is reabsorbed expanding the extracellular space and raising HCO_3^- concentration.

generation and K^+ and H^+ secretion by the distal tubule. The excess HCO_3^- generated produces the alkalosis (Fig. 4.6C). This type of alkalosis is maintained by the persistently high levels of mineralocorticoid and K^+ deficiency, both of which stimulate tubular $NaHCO_3$ reabsorption (Table 4.3).

Patients who develop alkalosis through mineralocorticoid excess, **since they have no prior volume or Cl^- deficits, have Cl^- in the urine in amounts commensurate with dietary intake.** With increased renal retention of Na^+, mild volume overload occurs, producing hypertension without edema.

In summary, the differential diagnosis of metabolic alkalosis may be divided into those **disorders with Cl^-** and those **disorders without Cl^- in the urine.** This can be seen in Table 4.2.

Clinical Features

The symptoms of metabolic alkalosis are **usually** due to the underlying disorder, hypokalemia, volume depletion or volume overload, and are not due to the alkalosis per se. Rarely, with severe alkalemia, there are symptoms of paresthesiae, carpopedal spasm and light-headedness which are related, at least in part, to increased cerebrospinal fluid pH.

One problem that can occur in patients with severe metabolic alkalosis and underlying chronic lung disease is worth emphasizing. Respiratory compensation for metabolic alkalosis leads to hypoventilation resulting in hypercapnia. Since patients with severe chronic lung disease often have borderline oxygenation, severe metabolic alkalosis can result in worsening hypercapnia, hypoxemia and respiratory failure.

Treatment

Treatment of metabolic alkalosis should initially involve correction of the underlying disorder, if possible.

For those disorders associated with low urine Cl^-, administration of Cl^-, either as the K^+ or Na^+ salt, will allow tubular reabsorption of a relatively higher fraction of Na^+ with Cl^-. This will correct the volume deficit, which will reduce aldosterone levels and tubular $NaHCO_3$ reabsorption leading to bicarbonaturia and correction of the alkalosis.

Excessive K^+ secretion will also cease. **The urine will remain Cl^- free until the Cl^- deficit has been corrected.** The effectiveness of NaCl in correcting the alkalosis leads some to categorize metabolic alkalosis with low urine Cl^- as **saline responsive.**

> In the case of metabolic alkalosis complicated by renal failure, HCO_3^- cannot be excreted in the urine and the alkalosis can only be corrected by providing H^+ (as NH_4Cl, HCl or arginine hydrochloride) or by dialysis against a low HCO_3^-, high Cl^- dialysate. Alkalosis in this setting is frequently due to vomiting or nasogastric drainage and can sometimes be ameliorated by administration of a histaminic H_2 receptor blocking drug (cimetidine, ranitidine) which inhibits gastric acid secretion. Also, aggressive K^+ replacement in the hypokalemic patient may help to correct the alkalosis by shifting K^+ into and H^+ out of cells in this setting.
>
> In the case of patients with metabolic alkalosis and low urine Cl^- but with total body Na^+ overload (e.g. patients with severe congestive heart failure who are on diuretics), saline would worsen the hypervolemia. Carbonic anhydrase inhibitors will inhibit HCO_3^- reabsorption in the proximal tubule, leading to bicarbonaturia, and, therefore, may sometimes be very helpful.

In patients whose primary event is increased tubular HCO_3^- generation, e.g. primary aldosteronism, Cl^- is present in the urine, there is mild volume expansion, **frequently with hypertension,** and the alkalosis is not corrected by Cl^- administration (leading some to categorize these patients as being **saline resistant**). Large doses of an aldosterone antagonist and K^+ replacement can correct this type of alkalosis.

With severe alkalemia (pH >7.60) one may see respiratory failure attributable to the compensatory hypoventilation (see above) or severe neuromuscular symptoms. Prompt treatment is indicated. Fortunately, infusion of HCl is rarely necessary.

Respiratory Acidosis

As previously defined, respiratory acidosis is caused by any alteration which causes a **primary increase in pCO_2.**

Etiology

The most important etiologies of respiratory acidosis appear in Table 4.4.

Pathophysiology

As discussed previously, the pCO_2 is determined by the balance between metabolic CO_2 production, which is relatively constant, and ventilation, which can vary rapidly over a wide range in response to a variety of factors. Respiratory acidosis occurs as a result of **hypoventilation.** When respiratory function is disturbed, pCO_2 rises, and uncompensated respiratory acidosis occurs: for example, H^+ concentration = 70 nEq/L, HCO_3^- concentration = 24 mEq/L, pCO_2 = 70 mm Hg.

Integrated Response to Respiratory Acidosis

The body reacts to the elevation of pCO_2 with a three-phase "defensive" response.

Buffering. First, a slight, but measurable increase in HCO_3^- concentration takes place immediately, due to chemical buffering. Bicarbonate, the principal extracellular buffer, can not take part in buffering CO_2, so that 97% of the acid load is buffered intracellularly and only

Table 4.4.
Principle Causes of Respiratory Acidosis

---

1. Inhibition of respiratory center
   A. Drug overdose: opiates, etc.
   B. Oxygen therapy in chronic hypercapnia
II. Musculoskeletal disorders
   A. Muscle weakness, e.g., myasthenia gravis
   B. Extreme obesity
   C. Chest cage abnormalities, e.g., kyphoscoliosis
III. Airway obstruction
   A. Aspiration of foreign body
   B. Asthma
   C. Chronic obstructive lung disease
IV. Abnormal pulmonary capillary gas exchange
   A. Pulmonary edema
   B. Severe lung disease
V. Inadequate mechanical ventilation

3% extracellularly. This results in a very slight increase in plasma HCO_3^- concentration.

> This increase in HCO_3^- concentration is about 1–2 mEq/L for every 10 mm Hg increase in pCO_2 above normal (normal = 40 mm Hg). Alternatively, the change in arterial H^+ concentration from normal is about 80% of the change in pCO_2 from normal. For example, H^+ concentration = 62 nEq/L, HCO_3^- concentration = 28 mEq/L, pCO_2 = 70 mm Hg.

Renal Compensation. Second, the increased pCO_2 and acidosis induce renal tubular cells to increase acid excretion, which is equivalent to increasing HCO_3^- generation. **Over a period of several days,** plasma HCO_3^- concentration will increase. Again, this metabolic compensation is **not sufficient** to restore the normal ratio of H_2CO_3 to HCO_3^-.

> Typically, plasma HCO_3^- concentration will increase by about 3–4 mEq/L for every 10 mm Hg increase in pCO_2 above normal. Alternatively, the change in arterial H^+ concentration from normal is about 30% of the change in pCO_2 from normal. For example, H^+ concentration = 49 nEq/L, HCO_3^- concentration = 34 mEq/L, pCO_2 = 70 mm Hg. **Bicarbonate concentration seldom is higher than 35 mEq/L** as a result of compensation for respiratory acidosis because patients rarely have a pCO_2 >65–70 mm Hg on a chronic basis.

Definitive Correction. The final restoration of normal acid-base homeostasis can be achieved under these circumstances only by an improvement of ventilatory function and restoration of pCO_2 to normal.

Clinical Features

The symptoms of **acute** respiratory acidosis are much more prominent than those of **chronic** respiratory acidosis and consist of a variety of neurologic symptoms progressing to somnolence and coma **(CO_2 narcosis).** CSF pressure may be elevated and papilledema can be seen on examination. This is probably due to increased cerebral blood flow seen in respiratory acidosis. With severe **acidemia** (pH <7.15) there is reduced cardiac contractility, peripheral vasodilation and release of endogenous catecholamines, frequently resulting in cardiac arrhythmias.

Chronic respiratory acidosis is frequently associated with cor pulmonale and peripheral edema. The cor pulmonale is due to chronic hypoxemia and the underlying lung disorder. The etiology of the edema may be the increased renal $NaHCO_3$ reabsorption which occurs as a compensatory mechanism in respiratory acidosis.

Treatment

Treatment of respiratory acidosis should first involve correction of the underlying cause, if possible. Bicarbonate administration should be avoided as this may raise cerebral interstitial pH and result in further depression of ventilation (cerebral interstitial pH is the major determinant of ventilation).

Respiratory Alkalosis

As previously stated, respiratory alkalosis is the result of any disorder which causes a **primary decrease in pCO_2.** It is one of the most common acid-base disorders.

Table 4.5.
Principal Causes of Respiratory Alkalosis

I.   Hypoxemia
   A. Congestive heart failure
   B. Pneumonia
   C. Pulmonary emboli
   D. High altitude
II. Pulmonary disease
III. Stimulation of respiratory center
   A. Salicylate intoxication
   B. Sepsis
   C. Psychogenic hyperventilation
   D. Brain lesions
IV. "Excessive" mechanical ventilation

Etiology

Table 4.5 shows the main causes of respiratory alkalosis.

Pathophysiology

By analogy with respiratory acidosis, respiratory alkalosis occurs as a result of **hyperventilation.** Reduced CO_2 production cannot cause reduced pCO_2 because basal CO_2 production is relatively fixed.

Integrated Response to Respiratory Alkalosis

This involves buffering, renal compensation and, finally, correction of the underlying disturbance.

Buffering. Ninety-nine percent of the alkali load in acute respiratory alkalosis is **buffered** intracellularly, largely by movement of H^+ out of cells resulting in a slight decrease in plasma HCO_3^- concentration.

> The decrease in HCO_3^- concentration is about 2.5 mEq/L for each 10 mm Hg decline in pCO_2. Alternatively, the change in arterial H^+ concentration from normal is about 80% of the change in pCO_2 from normal. The plasma HCO_3^- concentration rarely is less than 18 mEq/L as a result of buffering.

Renal Compensation. This occurs as result of a reduction in tubular $NaHCO_3$ reabsorption and requires 3–4 days to be fully manifest.

> This results in a **total decline** of plasma HCO_3^- concentration of about 5 mEq/L from normal for every 10 mm Hg decline of pCO_2 from normal in **chronic respiratory alkalosis.** It should be remembered, however, **that plasma HCO_3^- concentration rarely is below 15 mEq/L.** If this is the case, one should suspect superimposed metabolic acidosis.

Definitive Correction. Correction of the respiratory alkalosis requires correction of the underlying cause. It should be remembered, however, that full correction of the plasma HCO_3^- concentration back to normal is dependent on renal acid excretion and may require several days. During this time the patient may have a picture indistinguishable from metabolic acidosis (so-called **posthypocapneic metabolic acidosis**).

Clinical Features

The symptoms produced by **severe respiratory alkalosis** are primarily neurologic and include light-headedness, altered consciousness, paresthesiae, cramps, carpopedal spasm indistinguishable from that seen with hypocalcemia and syncope. Cardiac arrhythmias may also occur and can even result in death. It is felt that these symptoms are related to elevated CSF pH and to an effect of alkalosis on membrane excitability. In addition, severe alkalosis can reduce cerebral blood flow dramatically and this may contribute to the neurologic symptoms. Because of metabolic compensation (reduced plasma HCO_3^- concentration) which occurs over several days and results in a reduction of CSF pH toward normal, the more severe symptoms are not generally seen in **chronic respiratory alkalosis.**

Treatment

Treatment is solely directed at diagnosing and correcting the underlying disorder. With severe cardiac abnormalities or neurologic symptoms, a rebreathing mask or sedation may be required but this is unusual.

Complex Alterations of Acid-Base Homeostasis

The presence of two or more primary alterations in acid-base balance may give rise to complex and sometimes insoluble diagnostic problems.

It is relatively easy to uncover the presence of a **double alteration** (e.g. double alkalosis, with concomitant respiratory and metabolic alkalosis; or double acidosis), because of the obvious lack of compensation of the pCO_2 or HCO_3^- values to the primary alteration. For example, in primary metabolic alkalosis, pCO_2 should be higher than normal. If it is either normal or lower, one must suspect the concurrent presence of respiratory alkalosis.

It is more difficult to uncover and correctly diagnose **combined alterations.** For example, in a patient who has moderate metabolic acidosis and concurrent severe respiratory alkalosis, pCO_2 will be lower than expected for the level of HCO_3^- and H^+ concentration or pH can be in the normal or alkaline range. Under these circumstances it may be impossible to detect the presence of metabolic acidosis, since a chronic respiratory alkalosis itself can lower HCO_3^- concentration, unless the acidosis happens to be of the variety with an increased anion gap. In this case, the high anion gap will be a "tipoff" to the presence of this problem. A similar problem occurs when metabolic alkalosis is present with respiratory acidosis. In an effort to help in diagnosing such combined and double alterations and even more complicated combinations, the known relationship between the various primary alterations and their respective compensatory changes, as well as the clinical history, must be used. Thus, if the apparent compensation is above or below the degree of compensation expected for a given disorder, a combined alteration is suggested (see below).

Summary of "Expected" Compensation for Primary Acid-Base Disorders

METABOLIC DISORDERS
ACIDOSIS: $\Delta pCO_2 \cong (1.2 \pm .3) (\Delta HCO_3^-)$
NOTE: Acute compensation > chronic
ALKALOSIS: $\Delta pCO_2 \cong (0.7 \pm 0.2) (\Delta HCO_3^-)$
NOTE: pCO_2 usually not >55 mm Hg
RESPIRATORY DISORDERS
ACIDOSIS:
Acute: $\Delta HCO_3^- \cong (.1-.2)(\Delta pCO_2)$
$\Delta H^+ \cong 0.8 \Delta pCO_2$
Chronic: $\Delta HCO_3^- \cong (.3-.4)(\Delta pCO_2)$
$\Delta H^+ \cong 0.3 \Delta pCO_2$
NOTE: HCO_3^- is usually not > 35 mEq/L
ALKALOSIS:
Acute: $\Delta HCO_3 \cong 0.25 \Delta pCO_2$
$\Delta H^+ \cong 0.8 \Delta pCO_2$
NOTE: HCO_3^- is usually not < 18 mEq/L.
Chronic: $\Delta HCO_3^- \cong 0.5 \Delta pCO_2$
NOTE: HCO_3^- is usually not < 15 mEq/L

Suggested Readings

Cohen JJ, Kassirer, JP, Gennari FJ, Harrington JT, Madias NE. Acid-base. Boston: Little Brown & Company, 1982:113–376.

Kaehny WD. Pathogenesis and management of respiratory and mixed acid-base disorders. In: Schrier RW, ed. Renal and electrolyte disorders. Boston: Little Brown & Company, 3rd ed., 1986:187–206.

Kaehny WD, Gabow PA. Pathogenesis and management of metabolic acidosis and alkalosis. In: Schrier RW, ed. Renal and electrolyte disorders. Boston: Little Brown & Company, 3rd ed., 1986:141–186.

Pitts RF. Physiology of the Kidney and Body Fluids. Chicago: Year Book Medical Publishers, 3rd ed., 1974:162–212.

Rose BD. Clinical Physiology of Acid-Base and Electrolyte Disorders. New York: McGraw-Hill, 2nd ed., 1984:202–247 and 361–373.

ACID-BASE PROBLEMS

1. A 2-year-old boy is admitted to the hospital because of failure to thrive. In the course of his workup, he is found to have a blood pH of 7.32 and plasma concentrations of HCO_3^- 15 mEq/L, Na^+ 136, K^+ 3.1, and Cl^- 112 mEq/L.

   A. The acid-base disorder is:
      a. Metabolic acidosis with an elevated anion gap
      b. Metabolic acidosis with a normal anion gap
      c. Metabolic alkalosis
      d. Respiratory acidosis
      e. Respiratory alkalosis

   B. Serum phosphate concentration is low; blood glucose concentration is normal. The urine pH is 5.9; urine glucose test is positive. Which of the following is the most likely diagnosis?
      a. Fanconi's syndrome
      b. Diarrhea
      c. Asthma
      d. Renal tubular acidosis, distal variety
      e. Salicylate intoxication
      f. Aspiration of a foreign body

2. A 63-year-old patient with a history of chronic cough, dyspnea and edema is found to have the following plasma electrolyte concentrations: Na^+ 136, K^+ 3.6, Cl^- 89 and HCO_3^- 34 mEq/L.

   A. What alteration(s) in H^+ homeostasis could account for this picture? (Choose **all** that are correct.)
      a. Metabolic acidosis with an elevated anion gap
      b. Metabolic acidosis with a normal anion gap
      c. Metabolic alkalosis
      d. Respiratory acidosis
      e. Respiratory alkalosis

   B. What one test would be most helpful in pinpointing the acid-base disorder?
   - a. Urine Cl^- concentration
   - b. Serum lactate concentration
   - c. Plasma pCO_2 or pH
   - d. Plasma pO_2
   - e. Urine pH
3. If H_2SO_4 is produced by metabolism of dietary protein about 42% will be buffered by $NaHCO_3$ in the extracellular space.
   - A. What are the three end products of this buffering reaction?
   - B. Assume that the extracellular space is 10 L with concentrations in mEq/L of Na^+ of 140, Cl^- 104 and HCO_3^- 24. Following the production of 100 mEq H_2SO_4, how much is buffered in the extracellular space?
   - C. After the buffering reaction what are final concentrations of Na^+, Cl^- and HCO_3^- in the extracellular fluid?
   - D. How much change, if any, will there be in the anion gap?
4. An elderly gentleman presents to the accident room complaining of severe weakness and confusion. Blood pressure is 190/105 mm Hg. An adequate history cannot be obtained. Laboratory studies show plasma pCO_2 56 mm Hg, plasma concentration of HCO_3^- 42, Na^+ 144, K^+ 2.6 and Cl^- 82 mEq/L.
   - A. Calculate the H^+ concentration.
   - B. From straight line relation between pH and H^+ concentration, estimate the pH.
   - C. The following additional data are obtained: Scr 1 mg/dl, BUN 10 mg/dl and urine concentration of Na^+ 80, K^+ 40, Cl^- 90 and HCO_3^- <1 mEq/L. These data could be consistent with which **one** of the following possibilities?
     - a. Vomiting
     - b. Posthypercapneic alkalosis
     - c. Overdose of opiates
     - d. Primary aldosteronism
     - e. Severe emphysema
   - D. You stop all of the patient's medications. The next day the following data is obtained:
   Scr 1.1 mg/dl, BUN 9 mg/dl, and urine concentration of Na^+ 10, K^+ 25, Cl^- 2 and HCO_3^- <1 mEq/L. What diagnosis is this most compatible with?
5. Choose the corresponding pathophysiologic process from Column B for each cause of metabolic acidosis in Column A.

Column A	Column B
1. Diarrhea	a. Due to retention of H^+ and unmeasured anions normally produced by the diet
2. RTA	b. Often is complicated by respiratory alkalosis
3. Lactic acidosis	c. Excess acid usually produced due to tissue hypoxia from hypotension
4. Salicylates	d. Renal tubules secrete unidentified organic acids
5. Renal failure	e. Epithelial Cl^- (re)absorption causes hyperchloremia

6. A. What is pH if HCO_3^- concentration is 30.1 mEq/L and pCO_2 is 100 mm Hg? (Hint: Use the Hasselbalch variation of the Henderson equation.)

B. The acid-base disorder is :
   a. Metabolic acidosis with an elevated anion gap
   b. Metabolic acidosis with a normal anion gap
   c. Metabolic alkalosis
   d. Respiratory acidosis
   e. Respiratory alkalosis

C. Is it acute or chronic?

7. A 45-year-old man weighing 70 kg has acute gastrointestinal bleeding, followed by hypotension and confusion. He is noted to have labored breathing. Laboratory tests show plasma H^+ concentration 104 nEq/L, pH 6.97, pCO_2 12 mm Hg and plasma concentrations of HCO_3^- 3, Na^+ 140, K^+ 5.0 and Cl^- 104 mEq/L.

A. The acid-base disorder is:
   a. Metabolic acidosis with an elevated anion gap
   b. Metabolic acidosis with a normal anion gap
   c. Metabolic alkalosis
   d. Respiratory acidosis
   e. Respiratory alkalosis

B. Considering the clinical setting, what mechanism could be responsible for it?

C. Why is the patient laboring to breathe?

D. What is the appropriate therapy? Choose as many answers as are appropriate.
   a. Blood
   b. Intubation and mechanical ventilation
   c. Kayexalate

    d. $NaHCO_3$
    e. Oxygen
  E. How much?
    a. 735 mEq
    b. 245 mEq
    c. 25 G
    d. Enough to completely correct abnormality
    e. 3L per minute

8. A patient with glaucoma is taking acetazolamide to reduce intra-ocular pressure. He ingests a bottle of aspirin in a suicide attempt. Plasma tests show:

Na^+	K^+	Cl^-	HCO_3^-	pH	pCO_2
	(mEq/L)				(mm Hg)
140	3.8	116	12	7.40	20

  A. Characterize the acid-base disorder and give the cause.
  B. You give $NaHCO_3$; a few hours later tests show:

148	3.8	116	12	7.30	25

    Characterize this new acid-base disorder.
  C. What is responsible for the failure of $NaHCO_3$ to raise serum HCO_3^- concentration?
    a. The administered HCO_3^- is entering cells
    b. The administered HCO_3^- is entering the gut
    c. The administered HCO_3^- is consumed by newly produced acid
    d. The administered HCO_3^- is consumed by HCl
    e. The administered HCO_3^- is diluted out

9. A man with chronic lung disease is admitted to the hospital with superimposed pulmonary edema. Plasma test results show:

Na^+	K^+	Cl^-	HCO_3^-	pH	pCO_2
	(mEq/L)				(mm Hg)
139	4.2	100	30	7.37	54

  A. Characterize the acid-base disorder.

You order salt restriction and diuretics. He responds to treatment with a diuresis and resolution of pulmonary edema, but his breathing is more labored due to bronchoconstriction.

On Day 5 plasma tests show:

Na^+	K^+	Cl^-	HCO_3^-	pH	pCO_2
	(mEq/L)				(mm Hg)
136	3.8	86	40	7.32	80

    B. Characterize the acid-base disorder
    C. The patient is placed on a ventilator and the diuretics are stopped and after 3 days new tests show:

Na^+	K^+	Cl^-	HCO_3^-	pH	pCO_2
	(mEq/L)				(mm Hg)
129	3.6	82	37	7.53	46

      Characterize the acid-base disorder and give the cause.
    D. What is the appropriate therapy?
10. A 32-year-old man develops an acute upper gastrointestinal hemorrhage. During surgery, his blood pressure drops temporarily, causing acute renal failure. Following surgery he is severely oliguric; continuous nasogastric drainage is necessary because of evidence of persistent ileus. After 6 days, he is found to have the following set of plasma test results: pCO_2 54 mm Hg, Scr 8.6 mg/dl, and electrolyte concentration HCO_3^- 54, Na^+ 148, K^+ 4.9 and Cl^- 67 mEq/L.
    Characterize the two acid-base disorders and outline therapeutic modalities. (Hint: Take clinical setting and anion gap into account).
11. A 32-year-old woman has intrapartum hemorrhage and develops shock. Plasma tests show:

Na^+	K^+	Cl^-	HCO_3^-	pH	pCO_2
	(mEq/L)				(mm Hg)
140	5.0	102	6	7.15	18

A. Characterize the acid-base disorder and give the cause.
B. NaHCO₃ is administered and new tests with the patient still in shock show:

Na⁺	K⁺	Cl⁻	HCO₃⁻	pH	pCO₂
	(mEq/L)				(mm Hg)
150	4.9	99	15	7.35	28

Characterize the acid-base disorder.
The patient's blood pressure returns to normal after emergency surgery and blood replacement. New tests show:

Na⁺	K⁺	Cl⁻	HCO₃⁻	pH	pCO₂
	(mEq/L)				(mm Hg)
143	4.4	92	41	7.52	52

C. Characterize the acid-base disorder and give the cause.
12. A patient with severe diarrhea and chronic obstructive lung disease is admitted with the following laboratory values: pH 6.92, H⁺ concentration 120 nEq/L, pCO₂ 40 mm Hg and HCO₃⁻ concentration 8 mEq/L
   A. What are the two acid-base disorders?
   B. How could mechanical ventilation help the acid-base problem?

chapter 5

Potassium Disorders

David D. Clark

Elevated serum potassium (K^+) concentration, hyperkalemia, is seen in 1 to 10% of hospitalized patients and is frequently iatrogenic in nature. Reduced serum K^+ concentration, hypokalemia, can also be a complication of therapy and is seen in 20–30% of patients treated with thiazides, a commonly used group of diuretics. Fortunately, most of these abnormalities are mild and of no clinical importance. Nevertheless, severe disturbances of K^+ concentration may be life-threatening and consequently an understanding of the K^+ disorders is important for the clinician.

Physiologic Effects of Potassium

Total body K^+ is about 50–55 mEq/kg body weight. Potassium is the major cation in the intracellular fluid, where it has a concentration approximating that of extracellular Na^+ (as high as 150 mEq/L). The membrane enzyme, Na^+-K^+-ATPase, maintains the high intracellular concentration of K^+ and low concentration of Na^+ relative to the respective extracellular concentrations of 3.5–5.5 mEq/L and 135–145 mEq/L by transporting Na^+ out of and K^+ into cells in a 3:2 ratio. This pump works continuously, since both Na^+ and K^+ constantly leak down their respective concentration gradients into and out of the cell. Additionally, the outward diffusion of K^+ is opposed by the electrical affinity of K^+ for negatively charged intracellular proteins that cannot cross the cell membrane. The net result of these chemical and electrical forces is a charge separation across the cell membrane which produces the negative intracellular electrical potential of 90 mV relative to the outside of the cell **(transmembrane potential).**

Potassium and Cell Function

Potassium disturbances can have major effects on various cell functions and neuromuscular transmission. Potassium participates in the regulation of protein and glycogen synthesis and is required for normal responsiveness of renal tubular cells to ADH. In fact, patients with K^+ depletion have a reduced capacity to concentrate the urine and may develop polyuria. The depolarization of conducting and muscle cells also depends on normal levels of K^+ in the body.

Potassium and the Resting Membrane Potential

The **ratio** of the K^+ concentration within cells ($[K^+]_c$) to the K^+ concentration in the extracellular fluid ($[K^+]_e$) is the major determinant of the resting transmembrane potential **(Em)** as expressed by the formula:

$$\text{Em} = -61 \log \frac{r[K^+]_c + 0.01\,[Na^+]_c}{r[K^+]_e + 0.01\,[Na^+]_e} \qquad \text{equation 1}$$

where r is the $3:2$ active transport ratio of the Na^+-K^+-ATPase pump, 0.01 is the membrane permeability of Na^+ relative to K^+, and "c" and "e" refer to cellular and extracellular, respectively.

The resting transmembrane potential, in turn, is important in the generation of the action potential that is essential for normal neural and muscular function. The resting transmembrane potential is about -90 mV with the inside of the cell, as stated above, negative relative to the outside of the cell. When the transmembrane potential is more negative, the cell is said to be **hyperpolarized;** when the transmembrane potential is less negative or even positive, the cell is said to be **depolarized.** A depolarizing stimulus, if strong enough, reduces the absolute magnitude of the transmembrane potential above the **threshold potential, Et,** and an action potential propagates along nerve or muscle cells, resulting in neural transmission or muscular contraction (Fig. 5.1). Depolarizing stimuli of lesser magnitude, on the other hand, fail to elicit an action potential, if they do not depolarize the cell above

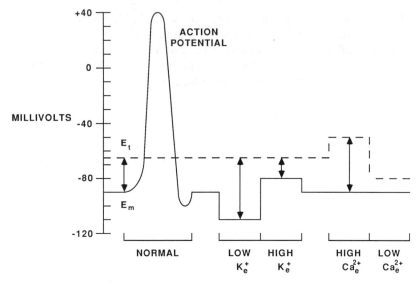

Figure 5.1.   Effect of extracellular K^+ and calcium concentrations on resting potential, Em, and threshold potential, Et. (Reproduced with permission from B.D. Rose, *Clinical Physiology of Acid-Base and Electrolyte Disorders,* 2nd ed., McGraw-Hill Co., New York, 1984).

the threshold potential. Thus, the difference between the resting trans-membrane potential and the threshold potential (Em-Et) determines the overall level of membrane excitability. Any factor which alters either potential, Em or Et, will alter the level of membrane excitability (Fig. 5.1).

Hypokalemia hyperpolarizes the cell. Hence, **Em-Et will be increased and the cell will be less excitable** (Fig. 5.1). An example of the clinical applicability of this fact is the flaccid muscle paralysis that can be seen with hypokalemia.

Conversely, **hyperkalemia** depolarizes the cell. Hence **Em-Et is decreased and the cell is more excitable.** With more severe degrees of hyperkalemia, however, the cell can actually be depolarized above the threshold potential. In this case the cell cannot repolarize after a single action potential (so-called **depolarization block.**) The clinical correlate of the latter phenomenon is also muscle paralysis.

It is important to realize that the **ratio** of intracellular to extracellular K^+ concentration determines the resting membrane potential. This may explain the observation that some patients with an extracellular K^+ concentration of 2 mEq/L on the basis of chronic losses of K^+ have few or no neuromuscular symptoms whereas other patients with acute hypokalemia of the same degree can be paralyzed. In **chronic** hypokalemia (e.g. diarrhea) depletion of the large intracellular pool of K^+ can reduce the impact of severe hypokalemia on Em. On the other hand, **acute** hypokalemia of similar magnitude caused by the translocation of K^+ into cells would cause greater hyperpolarization of the cell (e.g. hypokalemic periodic paralysis). Hence, the physiologic effect of hypokalemia, or hyperkalemia for that matter, may depend on the changes not only in extracellular but also in intracellular K^+ stores.

It is also important to appreciate that changes in the threshold potential, Et, can affect membrane excitability. The plasma Ca^{2+} concentration is of clinical relevance in this regard. **Hypocalcemia** increases the absolute magnitude of the Et (makes it more negative) and, hence, the term **Em-Et decreases and the membrane is more excitable** (Fig. 5.1). With **hypercalcemia,** the absolute magnitude of the Et is decreased, **Em-Et is increased and the membrane is less excitable.** This is important clinically because hypercalcemia tends to counteract the effect of hyperkalemia (**both** Em and Et change in the same direction and, hence, Em-Et is restored toward normal) and calcium salts are used in the treatment of severe hyperkalemia.

Regulation of Potassium Concentration

The extracellular K^+ concentration is regulated at 3.5–5 mEq/L in normal individuals. The total amount of K^+ in the entire extracellular space is only 50–80 mEq and approximates the daily intake of K^+ (60–120 mEq).

The small intestine readily absorbs dietary K^+. The maintenance of a "normal" serum K^+ concentration depends upon the ability of the numerous K^+ homeostatic systems to **balance** renal excretion of K^+ with intake and to adjust the **distribution** of K^+ between the intracellular and extracellular compartments. We will focus on the homeostatic mechanisms controlling balance and distribution separately. It should be realized, however, that these mechanisms work in concert, with mechanisms controlling distribution playing a more important role acutely, and mechanisms controlling balance playing a more important role chronically.

Homeostatic Mechanisms Affecting Potassium Distribution between Cells and Extracellular Fluid

A number of factors affect the distribution of K^+ between the intracellular and extracellular compartments. Physiologic factors protect the serum K^+ concentration from extreme elevation during K^+ loads such as eating and extreme depressions during K^+ losses such as acute diarrheal illnesses. Pathologic factors, on the other hand, may produce acute disturbances of K^+ distribution.

Physiologic Factors

The physiologic factors affecting K^+ distribution are listed in Table 5.1.

Plasma Potassium Concentration. Potassium loading leads to an elevation of plasma K^+ concentration and stimulates movement of K^+ into cells. Potassium depletion leads to reduced plasma K^+ concentration and results in movement of K^+ out of cells.

Catecholamines. β_2-adrenergic stimuli (mainly epinephrine) facilitate uptake of K^+ into cells. β_2-adrenergic blocking drugs (e.g. propranolol) **impair, but do not prevent,** cellular uptake of K^+ with K^+ loading. β_2-adrenergic stimuli, therefore, have a permissive role to play in the acute disposition of a K^+ load. On the other hand, at levels of catecholamines seen with extreme stress (e.g. myocardial infarction), plasma K^+ concentration may fall acutely by about 0.5–1.0 mEq/L.

Insulin. Insulin also promotes K^+ movement into cells and insulin deficiency impairs cellular uptake of K^+ during K^+ loading. As with β_2-adrenergic stimuli, the effect is an acute and permissive one more relevant to the disposition of a K^+ load rather than the maintenance

Table 5.1
Major Factors That Affect Transmembrane Movement of Potassium

Physiologic	Pathologic
Plasma $[K^+]$	Acidosis/alkalosis
Catecholamines	Cell breakdown/production
Insulin	Hyperosmolality
Na^+-K^+-ATPase	

of the steady state plasma K^+ concentration. With increased insulin levels K^+ movement into cells will be enhanced.

Na$^+$-K$^+$-ATPase. This is the major factor in maintaining a normal plasma K^+ concentration. Na$^+$-K$^+$-ATPase can be stimulated by insulin, catecholamines and aldosterone. Aldosterone is important in the enhanced cellular uptake of K^+ that occurs with chronic K^+ loading, perhaps via stimulation of Na$^+$-K$^+$-ATPase. However, the major effect of aldosterone on K^+ homeostasis is through its effect on renal K^+ excretion (see below).

Pathologic Factors

The pathologic factors affecting K^+ distribution are listed in Table 5.1.

Acidosis/Alkalosis. Metabolic alkalosis shifts K^+ into cells. Metabolic acidosis caused by inorganic (mineral) but not organic acids shifts K^+ out of cells due to the fate of intracellular H^+ and the need to maintain electroneutrality. For example, with metabolic acidosis due to administration of HC1, H^+ enters cells without Cl^- because Cl^- permeates cells poorly. Therefore, Na^+ or K^+ exit the cell in order to maintain electroneutrality. Lactic and other organic acids, on the other hand, also increase intracellular H^+ concentration, but the organic ion can enter the cell with the H^+ and electroneutrality is thus maintained without exchange of K^+ for the H^+. The reverse sequence occurs with metabolic alkalosis, but to a lesser degree than with metabolic acidosis. The changes in K^+ concentration with respiratory acid-base disturbances are relatively minor.

Cell Breakdown/Production. Cell breakdown (e.g. severe trauma, ischemia, catabolic states, etc.) causes release of large intracellular stores of K^+ and can result in hyperkalemia. On the other hand, situations associated with rapid cell production can result in cellular K^+ uptake and hypokalemia (e.g. patients with B_{12} deficiency who are given B_{12} and have a marked and immediate increase in production of red cells and platelets).

Hyperosmolality. Plasma K^+ concentration can rise with increases in effective osmolality (tonicity). Presumably water moves out of cells down the osmotic gradient and pulls K^+ with it into the extracellular space **(solvent drag).** An example of this phenomenon is the increase in plasma K^+ concentration seen with hyperglycemia.

Homeostatic Mechanisms Affecting Potassium Balance

Maintenance of K^+ balance depends on the kidney. While K^+ is freely filtered across the glomerular membrane, the great majority of this filtered K^+ is reabsorbed during passage through the proximal portions of the nephron such that only 5–10% is left in the urine by the distal tubule. This percentage of K^+ reaching the distal tubule remains constant under normal physiologic conditions. The variability of urinary K^+ excretion derives from the secretion of K^+ into the urine in the cortical collecting tubule. The movement of K^+ from the blood to the urine involves the active uptake of K^+ into the tubular cell and the passive movement of K^+ down an electrochemical gradient from the interior of the cell into the lumen of the tubule (K^+ secretion). The properties of the cortical collecting tubule cell which determine this passive movement of K^+ are depicted schematically in Figure 5.2. They are: 1) the negative transepithelial **potential difference** that favors movement of K^+ into the lumen, 2) the **chemical gradient** across the luminal membrane that favors movement of K^+ from the cell interior (high K^+ level) to the luminal fluid (low K^+ level), and 3) the K^+ **permeability** of the luminal membrane.

The four factors which can, in turn, influence these properties include: aldosterone, plasma K^+ concentration, tubular fluid flow rate, and Na^+ reabsorption without an accompanying anion (amount of impermeant anions) (Fig. 5.2).

Aldosterone. This increases the **permeability** of the luminal membrane of the cortical collecting tubule cell to K^+, and, as mentioned above, stimulates the activity of Na^+-K^+-ATPase on the peritubular side of the cell. The increased Na^+-K^+-ATPase activity enhances cellular K^+ concentration. Indirectly, the increased Na^+ reabsorption from the lumen enhances the electronegativity of the luminal membrane (see below). These latter two factors increase the **electrochemical** gradient favoring K^+ secretion into the urine. Adrenal production of aldosterone increases with K^+ loading (hyperkalemia) and decreases with K^+ depletion (hypokalemia) and thus aldosterone is a major physiologic regulator of K^+ balance.

Plasma Potassium Concentration. Plasma K^+ level directly affects the size of the K^+ transport pool (intracellular K^+), a major physiologic regulator of K^+ secretion and, hence, K^+ balance.

Tubular Fluid Flow Rate. Tubular fluid flow also influences this passive exit of K^+ by indirectly determining the luminal concentration

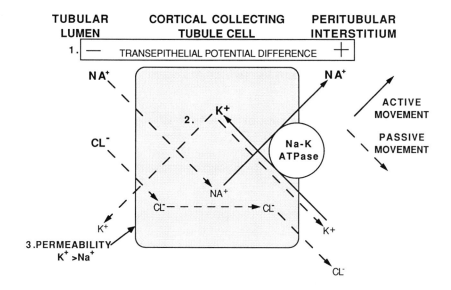

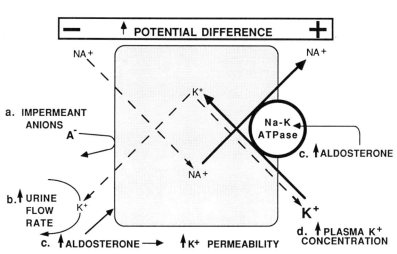

Figure 5.2. *Upper panel:* Schematic diagram of cortical collecting tubule cell showing the properties that contribute to the movement of K⁺ into the tubular lumen: (*1*) the transepithelial potential difference, (*2*) the chemical gradient of K⁺ concentration across the luminal membrane, and (*3*) luminal membrane permeability to K⁺. *Lower panel:* The factors that alter these properties in favor of K⁺ secretion include increases in (*a*) amount of impermeant anions, (*b*) urine flow, (*c*) aldosterone level, and (*d*) plasma K⁺ concentration. (Modified from B.D. Rose, *Clinical Physiology of Acid-Base and Electrolyte Disorders,* 2nd ed., McGraw-Hill Co., New York, 1984.)

of K^+ in the urine at this critical nephron site. When the flow rate is slow, the K^+ concentration builds up limiting the passive egress of K^+. A high flow rate facilitates the passive exit of K^+ by keeping the K^+ concentration in the urine low.

Sodium Reabsorption without an Accompanying Anion. The transepithelial potential difference at the site of K^+ secretion is oriented such that the lumen is negative, which facilitates K^+ and H^+ movement out of cells. Sodium reabsorption at this site, in turn, creates and maintains this favorable electrical gradient. When Na^+ is reabsorbed from the urine it leaves behind a slower moving Cl^-, which generates an electronegative transepithelial gradient. The transepithelial potential difference can be enhanced by the presence of an anion in association with Na^+ which is even less permeable than Cl^- (e.g. HCO_3^- in RTA, penicillins). Renal Na^+ avidity mediated by aldosterone will result in enhanced K^+ secretion in this situation. Otherwise, the anion will be excreted in the urine along with Na^+.

Hypokalemia

Definition

Ninety-five percent of individuals will have serum K^+ concentration of 3.5–5.0 mEq/L. Hypokalemia is, then, a serum K^+ concentration of less than 3.5 mEq/L.

Etiology

Vomiting, diarrhea and diuretics are the most common causes of hypokalemia. These and some other etiologies of low plasma K^+ levels are listed on Table 5.2.

Pathogenesis

In general, **acute hypokalemia** is a manifestation of an abnormality in one of the factors that enhances K^+ entry into cells (e.g. increased catecholamine activity).

> **Periodic paralysis** is a rare and poorly understood disease characterized by recurrent attacks of muscle paresis or paralysis. Attacks are thought to be due to sudden movement of K^+ into cells resulting in hyperpolarization of the cell mem-

Table 5.2.
The Principal Causes of Hypokalemia

I. Increased cell entry (acute)
   A. Catecholamines
   B. Insulin
   C. Alkalosis
   D. Production of new cells
   E. Periodic paralysis
II. Increased losses (chronic)
   A. Renal losses
      1. Primary mineralocorticoid excess (hypertensive)
         a. Endogenous
            i. Primary aldosteronism
            ii. Cushing's disease
         b. Exogenous
            i. High dose corticosteroid administration
            ii. Disorders simulating mineralocorticoid excess (licorice, tobacco)
      2. Secondary mineralocorticoid excess (normotensive)
         a. Vomiting, drainage from nasogastric tubes
         b. Diuretics
      3. Enhanced distal flow
         a. Diuretics
         b. Osmotic diuresis
      4. Na^+ reabsorption with a nonreabsorbable anion
         a. Penicillins
         b. HCO_3^- in RTA
         c. Ketones in diabetic ketoacidosis
   B. Extrarenal losses
      1. Gastrointestinal losses: biliary or pancreatic drainage tubes, fistulae, diarrhea
      2. Sweat losses
III. Reduced intake

brane and extreme weakness which can progress to paralysis and even death.

Chronic hypokalemia, on the other hand, reflects either renal or extrarenal loss of K^+.

If the loss is **renal** due to a change in one or more of the factors affecting K^+ balance (see above), urinary K^+ excretion will be inappropriately high for the low plasma level (>25 mEq/day or >15–20 mEq/L). This is most commonly due to diuretics which stimulate aldosterone secretion and increase distal flow. If the loss of K^+ is **extrarenal,** then urinary K^+ excretion will be low (<25 mEq/day or <15–20 mEq/L). This is most commonly due to diarrhea. In addition, chronic hypokalemia is almost always associated with either **metabolic alkalosis** (vomiting, mineralocorticoid excess, diuretics, etc.) or **acidosis** (diarrhea, RTA). For diagnostic purposes patients with **hypokalemia and metabolic alkalosis** can be further subdivided into those with and without chloride in the urine (see chapter on **acid-base disorders**) or those with hypertension (**primary** mineralocorticoid excess) and those without hypertension (**secondary** mineralocorticoid excess: vomiting, diuretics).

Since urinary K^+ excretion can be reduced to 10–25 mEq/day in response to K^+ depletion and normal dietary K^+ intake is 60–120 mEq/day, it is unusual to see K^+ depletion on the basis of reduced intake alone unless K^+ intake is severely and chronically limited.

Clinical Features

From the discussion of the physiologic effects of K^+ (see above), it can be appreciated that the major signs and symptoms of hypokalemia involve muscle and nervous tissues that are undergoing frequent depolarization. These include muscle weakness or paralysis (including intestinal ileus), cardiac arrhythmias (especially with digitalis), and EKG changes (Fig. 5.3). The main metabolic consequences of hypokalemia include interference with insulin release producing glucose intolerance and a nephropathy characterized by polyuria and polydipsia (nephrogenic diabetes insipidus).

Treatment

Treatment of hypokalemia depends on the magnitude of the estimated K^+ deficit and the severity of the clinical manifestations. Thus monitoring of the EKG and assessment of muscle strength is an essential first step in the management of hypokalemia.

Attempts should first be made to correct the underlying pathophysiology and stop ongoing K^+ losses, if possible. If the patient has mild-to-moderate hypokalemia (K^+ concentration = 2.8–3.5 mEq/L), is asymptomatic and is not on digitalis therapy need for K^+ supplements is controversial. However, oral replacement with KCl beginning at a rate of 60–80 mEq/day is considered appropriate by many physicians.

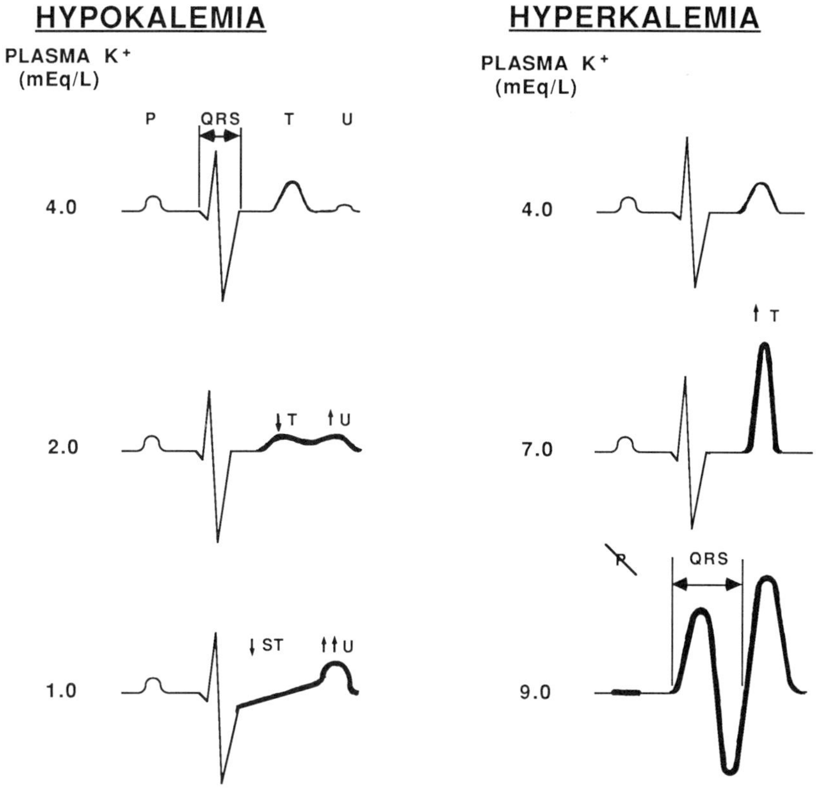

HYPOKALEMIA

PLASMA K⁺
(mEq/L)

HYPERKALEMIA

PLASMA K⁺
(mEq/L)

Figure 5.3. EKG changes in hypo- and hyperkalemia. As serum K^+ concentration **falls** the T wave becomes lower, flat or inverted while the U wave becomes taller. ST depression and arrhythmias may occur. As serum K^+ concentration **increases** the T wave becomes tall and peaked. With further rise the P wave decreases in height and disappears and the QRS and T waves widen. Eventually fusion and rounding of the QRS and T waves produces a sine wave. Ventricular standstill or fibrillation can occur.

With moderate-to-severe hypokalemia (K^+ concentration <2.8 mEq/ L), the patient will frequently remain asymptomatic but the K^+ deficits are larger and KCl can be given orally in larger doses. Regardless of the K^+ concentration, if the symptoms are severe and life-threatening (paralysis or cardiac arrhythmias), K^+ can be given intravenously at a maximum rate of 10–20 mEq/hour. The total amount of K^+ required to replete any deficit is unpredictable but the serum K^+ concentration may allow a rough estimate. In general, a decline in plasma K^+ concentration from 4.0 to 3.0 mEq/L correlates with a loss of about 200 mEq K^+ and a further decline of plasma K^+ concentration to 2.0 mEq/ L correlates with an additional loss of about 300 mEq K^+.

When treating hypokalemia, remember that the greatest risk is transient but potentially **life-threatening hyperkalemia** due to overzealous replacement; **plasma K^+ concentration and the EKG should be monitored frequently during vigorous replacement therapy.**

Hyperkalemia

Definition

Hyperkalemia is defined as a serum K^+ concentration greater than 5.0 mEq/L.

Etiology

The main causes of hyperkalemia are listed on Table 5.3. Renal failure and aldosterone deficiency are the most common etiologies, but in many patients act in concert with other causes.

Pathogenesis

The table lists some of the more common causes of hyperkalemia according to a pathophysiologic framework. **Pseudohyperkalemia** is due to movement of K^+ out of cells in the test tube as a result of an in vitro phenomenon. Hemolysis of blood entering a vacuum tube can release K^+ from red cells and produce an elevation of serum K^+ concentration. In addition, patients with high white blood cell counts ($>10^5$/mm^3) and platelet counts ($>5 \times 10^5$/mm^3) can release enough K^+ from the cells during blood clotting in the vacuum tube to raise *serum* levels. Measurement of a *plasma* (unclotted blood) K^+ concentration will correct for pseudohyperkalemia due to elevated white blood cell and platelet counts but not that due to hemolysis of blood entering the vacuum tube.

Acute transient hyperkalemia is usually due to movement of K^+ out of cells (abnormal K^+ *distribution*) or impaired uptake of a K^+ load produced by one of the physiologic or pathologic factors discussed earlier and listed on Table 5.3. On the other hand, **chronic** hyperkalemia is almost always associated with a defect in renal K^+ excretion (abnor-

Table 5.3.
Principal Causes of Hyperkalemia

I.   Movement out of cells (acute)
   A. Pseudohyperkalemia
     1. High platelet count
     2. High white blood cell count
     3. Hemolysis
   B. True hyperkalemia
     1. Catecholamine (β-adrenergic) blockade
     2. Insulin deficiency
     3. Acidosis
     4. Cell breakdown
     5. Hyperosmolality-hyperglycemia
II. Decreased urinary excretion (chronic)
   A. Renal failure (especially oliguric)
   B. Aldosterone deficiency
     1. Primary adrenal insufficiency
     2. Hyporeninemic hypoaldosteronism
     3. Inhibitors of aldosterone effect (K^+ sparing diuretics)
       a. Spironolactone
       b. Triamterene
       c. Amiloride
     4. Inhibitors of aldosterone production
       a. Angiotensin-converting enzyme inhibitors
       b. B_2 adrenergic blocking drugs
III. Increased intake

---

mal K^+ *balance*) due to advanced renal failure, hypoaldosteronism or both. Metabolic acidosis due to renal failure or hypoaldosteronism is also usually seen. One of the most common causes of hypoaldosteronism is **hyporeninemic hypoaldosteronism,** which often occurs in older diabetic individuals with mild renal insufficiency. These patients have low renin and aldosterone levels and, as a result, a defect in K^+ and H^+ secretion. Aldosterone deficiency can also be induced by a variety of drugs which either inhibit aldosterone effect or production.

Urinary K^+ excretion and cell K^+ uptake increase in response to acute K^+ loading. These protective responses are further enhanced with chronic K^+ loading in a process called K^+ **adaptation.** However, very rapid administration of K^+ (>160 mEq orally per dose), especially if given acutely, can result in transient and potentially fatal hyperkalemia. Usually, however, K^+ loads of this magnitude are not ingested in the course of ordinary daily life (normal dietary intake is

60–120 mEq/day). Hence, hyperkalemia due to chronic **excessive K^+ ingestion** is almost always seen in the presence of a defect in K^+ excretion.

Clinical Features

As with hypokalemia, the most prominent symptoms and signs of hyperkalemia involve depolarizing tissues and include cardiac (characteristic EKG changes and arrhythmias) and muscular (weakness, paralysis) manifestations. Hyperkalemia is often asymptomatic despite the EKG abnormalities until the occurrence of potentially fatal arrhythmias, including ventricular fibrillation or cardiac standstill. The typical EKG changes are outlined in Figure 5.3.

Treatment

Treatment should address the underlying abnormality, if possible, as well as the hyperkalemia itself. Since patients are frequently asymptomatic until they die from cardiac involvement, EKG monitoring, frequent assessment of muscle strength and frequent measurement of serum K^+ concentration are essential for patients with severe hyperkalemia (K^+ concentration >7 mEq/L.) Conversely, when serum K^+ concentration is less than 6 mEq/L, serious complications are rare. As with hypokalemia, the urgency and aggressiveness of therapy depend not only on the serum K^+ concentration but also on the clinical manifestations and EKG (Fig. 5.3).

The therapy of hyperkalemia includes the following measures:

a. **Counteracting the electrophysiologic abnormalities** with Ca^{2+} given intravenously (see Fig. 5.1). This is effective within minutes and should be given first with life-threatening manifestations but does not change body K^+ stores and must be given concurrently with measures that reduce body K^+ stores.

b. **Accelerating K^+ transfer into cells** with insulin (usually given with glucose to prevent hypoglycemia) and sodium bicarbonate intravenously. This is effective within an hour but does not change total body K^+. Measures to reduce total body K^+ stores must be given concurrently.

c. **Removal of K^+ from the body via the kidney** using furosemide or mineralocorticoid **or from the GI tract** using a K^+-binding resin (Kayexalate). Kayexalate is given with sorbitol to produce mild diarrhea. These measures are effective within hours and will reduce body K^+ stores.

d. **Removal of K^+ from the body via dialysis.** This is effective within hours and will reduce body K^+ stores (mainly used after failure of other techniques or with severe renal failure).

Suggested Readings

Knochel JP. Hypokalemia. Adv Intern Med 1984; 30:317–335.
Rose BD. Clinical Physiology of Acid-Base and Electrolyte Disorders. 2nd ed. New York: McGraw-Hill, 1984, Chapters 13, 26, 27, 28.
Williams ME, Rosa RM, Epstein RH. Hyperkalemia. Adv Intern Med 1986; 31:265–291.

POTASSIUM PROBLEMS

1. A 20-year-old nursing student is self-referred to you because of weakness. Examination is normal except for a weight that is 15% under normal for age and height. Serum electrolytes reveal Na^+ 138, K^+ 2.8, Cl^- 112 and HCO_3^- 14 mEq/L. Urine pH is 5.0. Blood pH is 7.30.
   A. The possible causes of the hypokalemia include (Choose **ALL** that apply.)
      a. Surreptitious use of diuretics
      b. Renal tubular acidosis
      c. Diarrhea induced by surreptitious laxative abuse
      d. Hypoaldosteronism
   B. Urinary K^+ excretion is 15 mEq/day. What is the diagnosis? (Choose **ONE** best answer.)
      a. Surreptitious use of diuretics
      b. Renal tubular acidosis
      c. Diarrhea induced by surreptitious laxative abuse
      d. Hypoaldosteronism
   C. What will happen to plasma K^+ if $NaHCO_3$ is administered to correct the acidosis? (Choose **ONE** best answer.)
      a. Increase
      b. Decrease
      c. Stay the same
2. A 17-year-old male is referred to your office because of persistent hypokalemia of 6 months' duration. He is a competitive wrestler and captain of his state champion high school team as well as a top student. On examination he appears healthy and has a slightly low blood pressure while standing. The serum electrolytes reveal Na^+ 140, K^+ 2.8, Cl^- 90 and HCO_3^- 38 mEq/L. Blood pH is 7.50.

   A. The possible causes of this picture include (Choose **ALL** that are applicable.)
     a. Surreptitious use of thiazide diuretics
     b. Habitual self-induced vomiting
     c. Hypoaldosteronism
     d. Hyperaldosteronism due to licorice abuse

   B. Urine chloride is 35 mEq/L. Which is the correct diagnosis? (Choose **ONE** best answer.)
     a. Surreptitious use of thiazide diuretics
     b. Habitual self-induced vomiting
     c. Hypoaldosteronism
     d. Hyperaldosteronism

3. A 28-year-old woman with insulin-dependent diabetes mellitus is admitted to the hospital with diabetic ketoacidosis, shock and stupor. Her laboratory data reveal: glucose 700 mg/dl, Na^+ 128, K^+ 5.7, Cl^- 85 and HCO_3^- 6 mEq/L. She is treated with insulin by continuous infusion and intravenous $NaHCO_3$ and NaCl without K^+ added because of the hyperkalemia and 12 hours later her laboratory data reveal: glucose 180 mg/dl, Na^+ 139, K^+ 2.2, Cl^- 102 and HCO_3^- 30 mEq/L.

   A. What were the total body stores of K^+ on admission? (Choose **ONE** best answer.)
     a. Increased
     b. Decreased
     c. Normal
     d. Cannot determine

   B. The factors that caused the plasma K^+ to be elevated on admission, include (Choose **ALL** that apply.)
     a. Release of K^+ due to excessive tissue catabolism
     b. Insulin deficiency
     c. Hyperglycemia
     d. Osmotic diuresis
     e. β_2 adrenergic stimulation
     f. Increased K^+ stores

   C. The factors responsible for the dramatic drop in plasma K^+ include (Choose **ALL** that apply.)
     a. Insulin therapy
     b. Reversal of excessive tissue catabolism
     c. Reversal of hyperglycemia
     d. Alkalosis

4. A 50-year-old male alcoholic is struck by a "hit-and-run" driver as he is walking down the street. He is found unconscious and with multiple trauma by a passerby, a nurse, who applies a tourniquet to his right thigh because of profuse bleeding from the lower extremity which does not stop with direct pressure. On arrival in the Emergency Room he is in shock and the right lower extremity is blue, cold and without a palpable pulse. He is given intravenous fluids and blood to correct his blood pressure and rushed to the Operating Room, where circulation to the right lower extremity is restored but the blood pressure remains low and he becomes anuric (no urine output). Serum electrolytes on transfer to the Intensive Care Unit reveal: Na^+ 140, K^+ 6.2, Cl^- 98 and HCO_3^- 12 mEq/L. Blood pH is 7.30.

A. Pathophysiologic factors involved in the development of acute hyperkalemia in this case include (Choose **ALL** that apply.)
   a. Lactic acidosis
   b. Tissue necrosis
   c. Oliguria
   d. β_2 adrenergic stimulation

B. Assuming the EKG is normal, the treatment of the hyperkalemia should involve all of the following **EXCEPT** (Choose one.)
   a. Restoration of blood pressure to reverse tissue ischemia
   b. Immediate dialysis
   c. Administration of $NaHCO_3$
   d. Administration of glucose and insulin
   e. Frequent monitoring of serum K^+ and the EKG

C. He remains in shock; the right lower extremity becomes more swollen and tender; the EKG reveals advanced life-threatening changes of hyperkalemia. He remains anuric. The plasma electrolytes reveal Na^+ 140, K^+ 8.8, Cl^- 88 and HCO_3^- 6 mEq/L. Blood pH is 7.14. The first thing to do is (Choose the **ONE** best answer.)
   a. start dialysis
   b. give Kayexalate and sorbitol
   c. administer $NaHCO_3$
   d. administer glucose and insulin
   e. give $CaCl_2$.

chapter 6

Glomerular Disorders

J. Gary Abuelo

The function of the glomeruli is to produce large quantities of plasma filtrate-free of cells and large proteins, but containing salts, water and metabolic wastes. As we will see in this chapter, a variety of immunologic, metabolic, hemodynamic and hereditary disorders may injure the glomeruli, permitting escape into the urine of red cells and albumin and reducing the GFR at times to levels incompatible with life. Patients with glomerular disorders tend to have one of three clinical syndromes, rather than a single typical illness. Some glomerular diseases mainly cause increased urinary red cells and renal insufficiency. They are said to have a **nephritic** clinical picture and are discussed under the section on **nephritic diseases.** Other conditions are chiefly characterized by leakage of protein across the glomerular capillary wall. They are said to have a **nephrotic** clinical picture and are discussed under the section on **nephrotic diseases.** Both nephritic and nephrotic diseases may fail to heal and may enter a stage characterized by slowly progressive damage that leads to total loss of renal function after several years. This will be discussed under the section on **chronic glomerulonephritis (GN).** An overview of the clinicopathologic features of the glomerular disorders is provided in Table 6.3 at the end of the chapter.

Nephritic Diseases

Definition

Nephritic diseases are glomerulopathies that may range greatly in clinical severity. Mild cases go unnoticed until a urine examination done for some reason shows increased numbers of red blood cells in the urine, visible only under the microscope. With greater disease activity, increased blood leaking through the glomeruli may make the urine red-tinged or even frankly bloody. Nephritic diseases may also impair glomerular filtration and cause azotemia and hypervolemia. The urine content of protein is usually only slightly to moderately increased.

Etiology

The nephritic diseases are traditionally classified into groups by their histologic appearance. Within each histopathologic group the various etiologies may in turn be categorized as either primarily renal or systemic conditions with secondary renal involvement. Table 6.1 lists the most important nephritic conditions according to this framework.

Pathogenesis

Most nephritic diseases are produced through immunological processes that involve either glomerular deposition of antibodies, i.e., immunoglobulins (humorally mediated injury) or infiltration with lymphocytes and macrophages (cellularly mediated injury).

Humorally Mediated Injury

Antibodies can deposit in the glomeruli in three ways:

They may be directed at an intrinsic glomerular antigen, such as the glomerular basement membrane (GBM). Anti-GBM antibodies directed against basement membrane collagen may be produced without any recognized antigenic stimulation and may deposit on the GBM, causing an **idiopathic crescentic GN,** or on the GBM and the alveolar basement membrane in the lungs, producing a GN and a hemorrhagic pneumonitis **(Goodpasture's syndrome).** The resultant immunoglobulin deposition on the glomerular and

Table 6.1.
Principal Causes of the Nephritic Syndrome

I.   Acute diffuse proliferative GN
     A. Poststreptococcal GN
     B. Other postinfectious GN
II. Focal proliferative GN
     A. Primary renal diseases
         1. IgA nephropathy (Berger's disease)
         2. Non-IgA forms
     B. Secondary renal diseases
         1. Lupus nephritis
         2. Polyarteritis nodosa
         3. Henoch-Schonlein purpura
         4. Nephritis of bacterial endocarditis
         5. Goodpasture's syndrome
III. Crescentic GN
     A. Primary renal diseases
         1. Idiopathic
         2. Acute diffuse proliferative GN
         3. Berger's disease (IgA nephropathy)
     B. Secondary renal diseases
         1. Lupus nephritis
         2. Polyarteritis nodosa
         3. Henoch-Schonlein purpura
         4. Nephritis of bacterial endocarditis
         5. Goodpasture's syndrome
IV. Alport's syndrome

alveolar BM may be stained with a fluorescein-labelled anti-IgG antibody, which produces a linear pattern by immuno-fluorescent microscopy.

Antibody may arise in response to a foreign antigen and may complex with that antigen in the circulation. The circulating immune (antigen-antibody) complexes produced deposit in the glomerulus. This process may occur in a variety of bacterial, viral and parasitic infections and produce GN. The most important examples of immune complex GN are those associated with streptococcal infections (**poststreptococcal GN**), **bacterial endocarditis,** hepatitis B virus and malaria. Autoantigens also may be involved, such as DNA in **systemic lupus erythematosus,** and tumor neoantigen in a variety of tumors. Circulating immune complexes deposit in masses in the mesangial areas or along the glomerular capillary walls. They may be seen with special stains by ordinary light microscopy, but are more easily detected either by electron microscopy or by immunofluorescent microscopy after staining kidney tissue with fluorescein-tagged anti-immunoglobulin antibodies. A granular pattern of deposition is observed. The majority of cases of human GN have no obvious infection or other recognized source of antigenic stimulation, but demonstrate such immune complex deposits and are also considered to be immune complex GN. Examples of this in man include **IgA nephropathy, Henoch-Schonlein purpura, membranous GN and membranoproliferative GN.**

An alternative mechanism of *in situ* formation has been proposed to explain glomerular deposition of immune complexes. According to this theory, antibodies are stimulated by an antigen, which itself has an affinity to deposit in the glomerulus. The antigen fixes in the glomerulus and subsequently this "planted antigen" is bound by antibody from the circulation. This planted antigen mechanism has been produced in animal experiments and may occur in some types of human GN now assumed to be caused by deposits of circulating immune complexes. Up until now, it has not been possible to prove that this mechanism occurs in human GN.

Cell-Mediated Injury

The evidence for cell-mediated GN in man is indirect. This type of process has been produced in chickens that were rendered incapable of mounting an antibody response with an immunosuppressive drug. When they were immunized with renal antigens, they developed a GN with inflammatory infiltrates but without immunoglobulin deposition. The frequent finding of human cases of **idiopathic crescentic GN** with absent or scant immunoglobulin deposition, but with infiltration by macrophages and some T lymphocytes has suggested a role for cell-mediated immunity.

Mechanisms of Injury

The manner by which immunoglobulins or inflammatory cells damage glomeruli varies from one form of GN to another and is only partly understood. In experimental forms of GN immunoglobulins bound to intrinsic glomerular antigens or to immune complexes fix complement. Some components of complement increase glomerular permeability to serum protein and lead to proteinuria, while other components are chemotactic factors for polymorphonuclear leukocytes, which then infiltrate the glomeruli. Macrophages also infiltrate the glomeruli, possibly as part of a cell-mediated immune response or possibly attracted by unknown chemotactic factors. These infiltrating cells release injurious lysosomal enzymes, such as collagenase, and reactive oxygen metabolites, such as hydrogen peroxide (H_2O_2), which attack the GBM and other structures. Recent evidence also suggests that prostaglandins released by these cells are important in mediating glomerular injury.

Human Examples of Immunologic Glomerulonephritis

In man **poststreptococcal GN** and the **nephritis of bacterial endocarditis** are characterized by deposition of bacterial antigen, antibody, complement and infiltrates of polymorphonuclear leukocytes and macrophages and, therefore, most closely resemble experimental models of immune injury.

In other forms of human GN only some features of this model pathogenetic mechanism are present. In **IgA nephropathy,** IgA and some complement are deposited in the mesangial areas, which undergo mesangial cell proliferation. An immune complex etiology involving the IgA class of antibodies is suggested by the finding of IgA deposition in normal appearing skin, elevated serum levels of IgA, and by the recurrence of this disease in normal kidneys transplanted into affected patients. There is, however, little, if any, polymorphonuclear infiltrate or obvious glomerular damage. In some cases of **crescentic GN,** there are no deposits of immunoglobulin or complement, but perhaps due to cell-mediated immunity one does find infiltrating monocytes and damage to the glomerular tuft. In other cases of crescentic GN the infiltrating cells may have been attracted by linear (anti-GBM antibody) or granular (immune complexes) deposits of immunoglobulin along the GBM accompanied by complement.

Crescent Formation

Crescentic GN is characterized by crescent formation, which is a cellular area in Bowman's space composed of fibrin, macrophages and proliferated epithelial cells, presum-

ably from the glomerular capillary wall and Bowman's cap-
sule. The cellular component of the crescent is thought to
arise as a response to the presence in Bowman's space of
fibrin that has leaked through a hole in the damaged glomerular capillary wall.

Alport's Syndrome

Some glomerulopathies are not immune mediated. For
example, in Alport's syndrome or hereditary nephritis there
is a genetic defect in GBM collagen synthesis. The GBM of
these patients is multilayered in some areas and extremely
thin in others. The specific biochemical nature of the collagen defect has not been identified.

Clinical Features

General Comments

Hematuria. Hematuria is thought to be caused by leakage of red
blood cells across the glomerular capillary wall. This assumption has
not been verified, since open holes in the glomeruli or red cells crossing
the capillary wall are almost never observed. However, one examines
such a tiny fraction of the glomerulus during routine electron microscopy that such holes might be easily missed.

Hematuria in the nephritic syndrome may be microscopic; i.e. the
urine appears normal to the eye, but has increased numbers of red
cells, when the pellet or sediment from a centrifuged sample is examined under the microscope. In gross hematuria of glomerular origin the
urine has a smoky translucency due to the red cells and a reddish
brown color (tea or Coca Cola color) due to the long exposure of hemoglobin to the acid pH of the urine. In contrast, hematuria from bleeding sources in the lower urinary tract has a bright red color.

Red Cell Casts. As the red cells proceed down the nephron some of
them may become encased in masses of protein that appear in the
urine in the cylindrical shape of the tubular lumen. These are called
red cell casts and are considered evidence for GN, although they may
rarely be seen in tubular or interstitial diseases.

Renal Failure. Reduced GFR is another common feature of the
nephritic syndrome. It is thought to be caused by endothelial cell swelling and polymorphonuclear leukocyte infiltration, which reduce surface area for filtration or reduce capillary wall permeability or both.
Reflex vasoconstriction of the pre- and postglomerular arterioles may

NORMAL

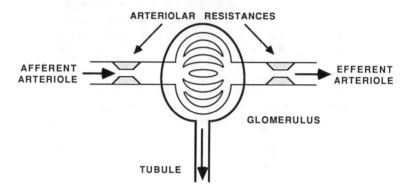

ACUTE NEPHRITIC SYNDROME

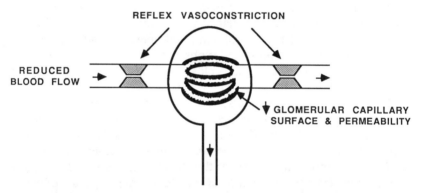

Figure 6.1. Mechanisms causing reduction of GFR in the nephritic syndrome. Diagram depicts arteriolar vasoconstriction and decreased ultrafiltration capacity of an affected glomerulus.

also contribute to reduced GFR by decreasing blood flow (Fig. 6.1). The fall in GFR can vary from mild, which produces asymptomatic azotemia, to severe, which leads to uremia or even total anuria.

Hypervolemia. Hypervolemia from incomplete urinary excretion of dietary Na^+ may be a feature of the nephritic syndrome. It can occur in patients with such reduced GFR that urine output has diminished to a few hundred milliliters per day or has completely ceased, but may also be seen in patients with only modest reduction of GFR. Clearly, the reduced renal Na^+ excretion is partly caused by reduced glomerular filtration of Na^+. However, for reasons that are not understood, reduction of tubular reabsorption of Na^+ does not operate effectively as a protective mechanism against hypervolemia. The manifestations of hypervolemia may vary in severity from mild peripheral edema to acute pulmonary edema or even malignant hypertension with encephalopathy (see chapter on **hypertension**).

Proteinuria. Immune-mediated glomerular injury increases glomerular permeability to serum proteins in all but the mildest cases of glomerulonephritis. The mechanism of increased permeability is not known with certainty, but it probably results in an increase in pore size and loss of fixed negative charge of the glomerular basement membrane. Thus, the glomerular capillary wall becomes generally more permeable to serum proteins, but particularly more permeable to negatively charged proteins, like albumin.

Proteinuria may be absent in some cases, even in the presence of gross hematuria. This paradox is explained by the fact that 1 ml of blood is enough to produce a red tinge when added to a liter of urine, but contains only about 36 mg of plasma proteins (0.6 ml plasma $\times$ 60 mg protein/ml plasma). The increase in protein content produced in the liter of urine is 3.6 ml/dl and is imperceptible in the clinical laboratory, where up to 15 mg/dl is considered normal.

Specific Conditions

Acute Diffuse Proliferative Glomerulonephritis. This is characterized by diffuse glomerular hypercellularity.

> Mesangial and endothelial cell proliferation and polymorphonuclear and monocytic infiltration are responsible for the cellularity. Granular deposits of complement and immunoglobulin are seen by immunofluorescence and electron microscopy in the mesangium and along the inside and outside surface of the GBM.

Eighty to 90% of patients have a previous history of a streptococcal sore throat or pyoderma (impetigo) 1–3 weeks before the onset of nephritis. Only certain strains of streptococci (nephritogenic strains) are associated with GN. There is evidence that these strains share a common intracellular antigen which has "nephritogenic" potential. In most cases one can document the previous streptococcal infection with culture or with serological tests. These tests detect antibodies in the patient's serum to streptococcal antigens such as streptolysin O, hyaluronidase and deoxyribonuclease B. In 10–20% of cases of acute diffuse proliferative GN there is no clinical or laboratory evidence for a streptococcal infection. While the etiology in these cases is usually unknown, occasionally there is a bacterial endocarditis, pneumococcal pneumonia or other acute infection associated with the GN.

Acute diffuse proliferative GN may produce the most typical and most severe cases of the nephritic syndrome. On the other hand, milder cases are far more common; microscopic hematuria with or without proteinuria may be the only manifestation.

Usually patients recover their renal function and have microscopic hematuria and low-grade proteinuria for several months. Rare patients with acute renal failure will not recover and will require dialysis. This may be associated with many crescents on the initial renal biopsy. Another rare outcome is for patients to progress to end stage renal disease after many years.

Focal Proliferative Glomerulonephritis. This is characterized by hypercellularity of some segments of some glomeruli.

> The immunoglobulin deposition observed depends on the specific disease. Mesangial IgA is characteristic of IgA nephropathy and Henoch-Schonlein purpura; mesangial IgG and complement with or without additional granular deposition along the GBM are seen in lupus nephritis and bacterial endocarditis; linear deposition of IgG along the GBM characterize Goodpasture's syndrome; and absent or traces of immunoglobulin are typical of polyarteritis nodosa.

Classically, **IgA nephropathy, Berger's disease,** presents as an episode of gross hematuria 1–3 days after an upper respiratory infection. One-half of affected patients will have one or several of these episodes occurring over years. Alternatively, other patients may just have asymptomatic urinary abnormalities, i.e. proteinuria or microscopic hematuria or both. On occasion, IgA nephropathy produces a full-blown nephritic syndrome. Most individuals with Berger's disease run a benign course which goes on for many years, although some 25% of cases eventually go on to chronic renal failure.

Non-IgA forms of primary focal proliferative GN have a variety of patterns on immunofluorescence from negative to mesangial deposition of immunoglobulins other than IgA or mesangial complement alone. Clinically they behave like IgA nephropathy.

Lupus nephritis will be discussed under nephrotic syndrome.

Polyarteritis nodosa produces narrowing or complete occlusion of small- and medium-sized blood vessels anywhere in the body. Ischemia or infarction in various locations leads to symptoms from multiple organ systems such as peripheral neuropathy, rash, gastrointestinal bleeding, myalgias and arthritis. Patients also have generalized symptoms such as fever, fatigue and weight loss. In the kidney, infarction due to involvement of medium-sized arteries may cause flank pain and gross hematuria. Even more common clinically, however, is a nephritic picture due to a focal proliferative GN. Worsening renal function is associated with evolution to a crescentic GN. Despite treatment with steroids and immunosuppressive drugs, about one-third of patients die and most of the survivors have chronic renal failure.

Henoch-Schonlein purpura is a syndrome of unknown etiology characterized by a *rash* over the extensor surfaces of the extremities with one or more of the following complications: *arthritis, hemorrhagic gastroenteritis and nephritis.* Areas of skin involved by the rash have IgA deposits. Clinically patients manifest an acute nephritic syndrome of variable severity, which usually goes on to resolve without sequellae, although progression to end stage may occur in patients who develop crescentic GN.

Nephritis of bacterial endocarditis is a focal GN which may complicate bacterial endocarditis. Clinically it presents a nephritic syndrome of variable severity. Splenomegaly is common. Extrarenal manifestations such as fever, weight loss, petechial rash and arthritis may suggest a vasculitis or systemic lupus erythematosus. The glomerular lesion usually resolves spontaneously with successful antibiotic treatment of the underlying endocarditis.

In **Goodpasture's syndrome** an antiglomerular basement membrane (anti-GBM) antibody produces a focal proliferative GN accompanied by massive pulmonary hemorrhage. Usually, the first symptom is recurrent hemoptysis and only after days or weeks does a nephritic picture of varying severity develop. Occasionally an acute nephritic syndrome appears first and pulmonary hemorrhage occurs after several weeks. In most cases the renal lesion progresses rapidly to crescent formation and total glomerular destruction, leading to uremia within a few weeks or months. Death may also result from pulmonary hemorrhage.

Crescentic Glomerulonephritis. This is characterized pathologically by the presence of crescents in more than 50% of the glomeruli and clinically by the rapid worsening of renal failure associated with the nephritic syndrome. It occurs as a primary (idiopathic) nephropathy in about half of patients, in whom it may be associated with either linear immunofluorescent staining for IgG (anti-GBM antibody), granular staining for immunoglobulin (an immune complex GN) or negative staining for immunoglobulin (? cell-mediated GN). In the other half of patients crescentic GN is secondary to an otherwise more benign form of GN which has taken a malignant course. Thus, crescentic GN is described in poststreptococcal GN, membranoproliferative GN and **all the diseases that produce focal proliferative GN.** Improvement in renal function can occur spontaneously in some patients or can be induced with large doses of steroids in others. In any case, anuria or crescents in more than 80–90% of glomeruli lower the chance of recovery.

> What all these nephritides have in common is that when they are particularly severe they cause local areas of necrosis of the glomerular tuft. A break occurs in the capillary wall, allowing spillage of whole blood into Bowman's space. This stimulates an influx of macrophages and proliferation of the epithelial cells of Bowman's capsule, resulting in the formation of a cellular crescent.

Alport's Syndrome. This is a condition usually inherited as an X-linked genetic defect in GBM collagen synthesis with reduced expression in the female. Electron microscopy shows characteristic areas of GBM that are very thin and other areas that are split or multilayered. After many years the glomeruli may develop chronic sclerotic changes. Patients manifest ocular, auditory and/or renal abnormalities. The ocular defects include myopia and other abnormalities of the lens. The auditory defect presents as high frequency nerve deafness. The renal abnormality begins clinically as hematuria and proteinuria. Many individuals, particularly women, have lifelong hematuria with little or no impairment of function, while others, particularly men, may gradually develop severe renal failure during their adult life.

Laboratory Features

Laboratory abnormalities in the nephritic syndrome include microscopic or gross hematuria with or without red cell casts, mild-to-moderate proteinuria and various degrees of azotemia. Low serum levels of total hemolytic complement activity and complement components, C3 and C4, may result from complement activation in some immune complex-mediated diseases. They are seen in about 90% of patients with acute diffuse proliferative GN or the nephritis of bacterial endocarditis, and also can occur in lupus nephritis and membranoproliferative GN, which will be discussed under the section on **nephrotic diseases.** High levels of antibodies against at least one streptococcal antigen are seen in over 90% of cases of poststreptococcal GN, and antistreptolysin O (ASLO), anti-DNase B, antihyaluronidase titers should be obtained in suspected cases.

Diagnosis

One may suspect the nephritic syndrome in any patient with hematuria and proteinuria. The presence of red cell casts or worsening azotemia make the diagnosis almost a certainty. In patients with poststreptococcal GN and GN caused by systemic disease, the etiology of the nephritic syndrome is usually apparent from the clinical picture, e.g. fever, heart murmur and positive blood culture in bacterial endocarditis. On the other hand, patients with a primary glomerular disease, such as idiopathic crescentic GN, require a renal biopsy for diagnosis.

Treatment

Antibiotics are used in bacterial endocarditis and poststreptococcal GN. Polyarteritis nodosa and Goodpasture's syndrome have been treated with corticosteroid and immunosuppressive agents, but the efficacy of these agents is inconsistent and uncertain. In addition, removal of the patient's plasma (plasmapheresis) in Goodpasture's syndrome reduces anti-GBM antibody levels and may prevent renal failure and improve pulmonary hemorrhage. Large doses of corticosteroids may stop the disease process in crescentic GN and permit improvement in renal function in cases with good urine output or crescents in <80% of glomeruli. Diuretics and salt restriction should be prescribed for the volume overload of the nephritic syndrome and dialysis for renal failure (see chapter on **acute renal failure**).

Nephrotic Diseases

Definitions

When patients with glomerular disease develop the **tetrad of heavy proteinuria, hypoalbuminemia, hyperlipidemia, and edema,** they are said to have the **nephrotic syndrome.** An increase in glomerular permeability with leakage of large amounts of protein into the urine is the primary defect. The other features of the syndrome develop secondarily. Although entitled nephrotic diseases, this section will actually discuss **heavy proteinuria,** its pathology, and its clinical manifestations.

Almost any kidney disease can increase urinary protein excretion above the normal limit of 150 mg/day. **However, heavy proteinuria with losses exceeding 3 gm/day is virtually always due to glomerular lesions rather than a tubulointerstitial or vascular renal disease.** This amount of proteinuria is in the same range as that seen in the nephrotic syndrome, and is, therefore, defined as **nephrotic range proteinuria** whether or not one has the full-blown clinical syndrome.

Etiology

Lipoid nephrosis accounts for about 90% of cases of nephrotic syndrome in preschool age children. This condition is less common in older individuals in whom other primary glomerulopathies and renal involvement by systemic diseases become prevalent. The most important etiologies of the nephrotic syndrome are listed on Table 6.2.

Pathogenesis

General Comments

When heavy proteinuria occurs, the glomerular "leak" mainly involves plasma proteins with molecular weights between 50,000 and 200,000 daltons. Albumin (MW 69,000 daltons) is the predominant protein in the urine of nephrotic patients, but in some cases IgG (MW 150,000 daltons) and other proteins in this molecular size range may also be lost in great enough quantities to cause clinical manifestations.

Table 6.2.
Principal Causes of the Nephrotic Syndrome

I. Systemic renal diseases
   A. Amyloidosis
   B. Diabetic glomerulosclerosis
   C. Lupus nephritis
II. Primary renal diseases
   A. Lipoid nephrosis
   B. Focal segmental glomerulosclerosis
   C. Membranous GN
   D. Membranoproliferative GN

Larger proteins such as IgM (MW 900,000 daltons) are usually retained normally by the glomerulus.

The defect responsible for glomerular leak of protein is an enigma. We might expect to see thinning or decreased density of the glomerular basement membrane to explain the increased permeability seen in nephrotic diseases. Alternatively we might expect defects in the slit diaphragms between the foot processes. Nothing of the kind is seen, however, when kidney biopsies from patients with nephrotic range proteinuria are examined by electron microscopy. The changes vary with the disease, but generally one sees a normal or thickened GBM and "fusion" of the foot processes with loss of slit diaphragms. These alterations would seem to be more compatible with decreased rather than increased permeability to plasma proteins. It is postulated that in some patients the glomerular capillary wall loses its fixed negative charge, which normally retards the passage of negatively charged albumin. This could greatly increase the clearance of albumin without producing defects visible on electron microscopy, and without greatly changing passage of IgG which is too large to pass through glomerular pores. In other individuals with significant losses of IgG and other larger proteins glomerular pore size is also thought to be increased. The reduced fixed negative charge and increased pore size responsible for proteinuria may come about through several different mechanisms. In no case, however, is the exact biochemical or structural defect known.

In some diseases physicochemical changes in a serum protein may contribute to proteinuria by facilitating the protein's passage through the glomerular capillary wall into the urine preferentially over the normal serum protein. In lipoid nephrosis, for example, an albumin with less negative charge and different conformation than normal appears in the serum and seems to play such a role. This altered albumin disappears when the patient's condition responds to treatment. In diabetes mellitus, glycosyl albumin may also be such a protein. It is produced by hyperglycemia through the irreversible covalent attachment of glucose to circulating albumin and exhibits enhanced transglomerular passage compared to the unglycosylated protein.

Specific Conditions

Amyloidosis. In amyloidosis there is infiltration of the GBM and other parts of the glomeruli with amyloid fibrils, of which there are two types. In one type seen with primary amyloidosis or amyloidosis due to multiple myeloma, amyloid protein forms from immunoglobulin light chains. In primary amyloidosis one frequently finds a monoclonal immunoglobulin in the serum or urine and moderate plasmacytosis in the bone marrow. Thus, primary amyloidosis is now thought to be due to a covert plasma cell disorder. In the other type seen with secondary amyloidosis, the amyloid is made up of a unique protein called AA protein, which is thought to derive from an antigenically related protein in the serum called SAA protein.

Diabetic Nephropathy. In diabetic nephropathy the hallmark of the glomerular changes is increased thickness of the GBM and mesangial matrix. It is thought that the metabolic abnormalities of diabetics lead to increased synthesis of these extracellular substances, but it is not known how this increases glomerular leakage of protein. Other evidence suggests that the GBM of diabetics may have reduced negative charges which would contribute to proteinuria. It has also been proposed that increased blood flow to diabetic glomeruli may also contribute to the pathogenesis of diabetic glomerulosclerosis (see chapter on **renal perfusion disorders**).

Lupus Nephritis, Membranous GN and Membranoproliferative GN. These are immune complex mediated forms of GN. In lupus nephritis, immune complexes consist in part of DNA and its antibody, which is easily detected in the serum. Focal proliferative, diffuse proliferative and membranous forms of immune complex GN are seen in SLE. In membranous and membranoproliferative GN patients usually have no associated extrarenal diseases and the specific antigens involved in the immune complexes are not known.

Exceptionally tumor antigens or hepatitis B antigen have been described in the glomeruli of patients with membranous GN secondary to malignancies or chronic hepatitis. Membranous GN may occur in patients with systemic lupus erythematosus. In some cases membranoproliferative GN has been associated with chronic hepatitis B or other infections. It is not certain how the glomerular leak of protein results from the presence of immunoglobulins, complement and in lupus nephritis polymorphonuclear and monocytic leukocytes in the glomeruli.

Lipoid Nephrosis. Patients with lipoid nephrosis develop severe proteinuria. It has been assumed that this is not an immunologically mediated condition because there are no inflammatory cells on histologic examination of their renal biopsies and their kidneys have no deposits of immunoglobulin and C'. Nevertheless, other observations suggest that this may, in fact, be an immunologic disease. These patients 1) frequently develop proteinuria shortly following a common cold, 2) often have abnormal immunoglobulin levels and 3) usually have a dramatic remission in proteinuria with corticosteroids or other immunosuppressive agents. A theory has been proposed that patients with this disease harbor a renegade population of lymphocytes. Under the influence of a viral infection of the upper respiratory tract the lymphocytes produce a lymphokine that increases glomerular capillary permeability to protein. It is speculated that treatment with immunosuppressive agents suppresses this clone of lymphocytes. It is hoped that future research efforts will shed some light on this hypothesis.

Focal Segmental Glomerulosclerosis. This may be a variant of lipoid nephrosis, since like lipoid nephrosis it may exacerbate after a cold and remit with corticosteroids. Also some cases of focal sclerosing GN develop in patients with lipoid nephrosis. The pathogenesis of focal sclerosing GN is unknown, although the disease often recurs in a kidney transplanted into an affected patient, suggesting that it is induced by circulating factors in the patient's plasma.

Clinical Features

General Comments

Heavy Proteinuria. Many patients with heavy proteinuria have no symptoms. The glomerular leak of albumin leads to a fall in serum albumin concentration insufficient to provoke clinical manifestations. The drop in albumin level stimulates increased synthesis by the liver and reduces overall albumin catabolism. Urinary albumin losses decrease because lower plasma concentrations are presented for filtration to the glomeruli. A new steady state is reached with increased synthesis and reduced breakdown, balancing out the urinary losses.

Edema. If protein losses increase the albumin pool of the body is further depleted, until reduced serum albumin levels and intravascular oncotic pressure lead to edema formation. This usually occurs when the daily protein losses exceed 3 gm and serum albumin is less than 3 gm/dl.

Hyperlipidemia. The low colloid osmotic pressure gives rise by unknown mechanisms to hyperlipidemia. Serum cholesterol, phospholipids and to a lesser degree triglycerides increase, as do levels of low density and very low density lipoproteins. As might be anticipated, the hyperlipidemia places patients with longstanding nephrotic syndrome at greater risk for **atherosclerosis,** which has even been seen in children with the nephrotic syndrome.

Bacterial Infections. Peritonitis, cellulitis or sepsis occur occasionally in patients with nephrotic syndrome. The presence of ascites might increase susceptibility to peritoneal infection. In addition, urinary losses of IgG and alternate pathway complement components may reduce host defenses against infection. In contrast, urinary losses of C3, C4 and other classical pathway complement components are not significant.

Thromboembolic Phenomena. The nephrotic syndrome may produce a hypercoaguable state with a tendency for thromboembolic phenomena. This is partly due to increased urinary losses of antithrombin III (MW 65,000). In addition the levels of several clotting factors increase by an unknown mechanism. Clinically, one may see arterial and venous thromboses and pulmonary emboli from peripheral veins. Partial renal vein thrombosis may also occur in as many as one-half of nephrotic patients. This usually causes no symptoms, but may be a source of pulmonary emboli or may obstruct venous outflow of the kidney.

Lipiduria. The glomerular leak in patients with heavy proteinuria usually produces lipiduria. Examination of the urinary sediment may show fat-filled tubular cells (oval fat bodies) or cholesterol crystals which form Maltese crosses in polarized light (doubly refractile fat bodies). Urinary lipid losses do not have any clinical significance.

Hematuria. Microscopic hematuria may be seen in any of the diseases that produce the nephrotic syndrome.

Hypertension. Increased blood pressure may be seen in any of the diseases that produce the nephrotic syndrome.

Nephritic Features. Membranoproliferative GN and the diffuse proliferative form of lupus nephritis may have gross hematuria, red cell casts, reduced GFR and hypervolemia in addition to a nephrotic picture.

Specific Conditions

Renal Amyloidosis. This is characterized by amyloid deposits in the glomeruli and elsewhere in the kidney. It usually begins after the age of 40, except in the face of a known cause such as chronic osteomyelitis. Most patients present with nephrotic range proteinuria or frank nephrotic syndrome, while others manifest moderate proteinuria. Patients with renal amyloidosis usually have continued nephrotic syndrome and progress to end stage renal failure. Death can also be due to amyloid involvement of other organs especially the heart.

Diabetes Mellitus. This may produce papillary necrosis and pyelonephritis; however, the most important diabetic lesion is intercapillary glomerulosclerosis: thickening of the GBM and overproduction of mesangial matrix. The mesangial areas may widen to a nodular appearance typical of nodular glomerulosclerosis (Kimmelstiel-Wilson disease). Diabetic glomerulosclerosis or nephropathy occurs mostly in patients with insulin-dependent diabetes for at least 10 or 15 years. The "triopathy," diabetic nephropathy, **retinopathy** and **neuropathy,** are frequently found together in patients and are considered complications of the generalized microangiopathy of diabetes mellitus. In particular, patients with renal disease **almost invariably** have simultaneous diabetic retinopathy. The first sign of diabetic glomerulosclerosis is proteinuria, which increases after months to years and gives rise to the nephrotic syndrome. Then renal function progressively deteriorates, leading within a few years to severe renal failure. Control of hypertension may slow the course of the renal disease. There is no good evidence that careful control of diabetes protects against the development or progression of the glomerular lesion.

Lupus Nephritis. This occurs in some 50–75% of patients with systemic lupus erythematosus, usually when their disease is active. The antinuclear antibody test (ANA) is positive and often complement levels are low. Renal involvement may be manifested clinically as a symptomless proteinuria which remains unchanged for months or years (typically focal proliferative form), as nephrotic syndrome (membranous or diffuse proliferative forms) or as a severe nephritic syndrome (diffuse proliferative form). Patients with focal proliferative and membranous GN do not often progress to chronic renal failure. Focal proliferative and diffuse proliferative lupus GN may respond to steroids. If renal failure does not improve with steroids, steady progression to renal failure often ensues. Various cytotoxic drugs, such as cyclophosphamide have also been used, but evidence for their effectiveness is preliminary.

Lipoid Nephrosis. This is also known as minimal change disease because its appearance on light microscopy is normal or nearly so. There are no immune deposits and electron microscopy shows only foot process fusion. It is responsible for most of the nephrotic syndrome occurring in children less than 5 years old, but only for a minority of nephrotic syndrome occurring in adults. The usual clinical picture is the sudden onset of nephrotic syndrome. In one-third of cases this follows an upper respiratory infection by a few days. Most patients will respond to prednisone after 2–4 weeks with a dramatic remission of their proteinuria. Unfortunately, most steroid-responsive patients will eventually relapse and follow the characteristic course of having one to many relapses, all steroid responsive, occurring over years with eventual cure and no residual renal impairment. Cyclophosphamide, a cytotoxic drug used to treat cancer, has been employed successfully in patients with lipoid nephrosis to induce permanent remission or to delay relapse for a year or more. Since cyclophosphamide therapy has serious complications, its use is generally limited to patients who have developed intolerable side effects of steroids.

Focal Segmental Glomerulosclerosis. This is also known as focal sclerosing GN and is characterized by focal and segmental sclerosis and hyalinosis. It is the cause of a minority of the cases of nephrotic syndrome seen in children and adults. The usual clinical picture is that of nephrotic syndrome. Corticosteroids may induce a remission in up to one-fourth of patients. Frequent steroid-sensitive relapses usually occur. Most steroid nonresponsive patients follow a clinical course of nephrotic syndrome unaffected by treatment and ending with the gradual progression to chronic renal failure. This disease may also present as asymptomatic proteinuria or chronic renal failure. Focal segmental glomerulosclerosis can recur in a renal transplant.

Membranous Glomerulonephritis. This disease is characterized by subepithelial immune complex deposits and thickening of the GBM by spike formation. It is one of the most common causes of adult nephrotic syndrome and occasionally occurs in children. The majority of patients have a nephrotic syndrome unresponsive to steroids. The disease follows an extremely variable course with as many as 25% of patients going on to a clinical cure, 50% of the patients continuing to have nephrotic syndrome or proteinuria and 25% of the patients progressing to chronic renal failure after 8–10 years of disease. Treatment with corticosteroids and immunosuppressive agents is controversial.

Membranoproliferative Glomerulonephritis. This glomerulopathy is characterized by subendothelial immune complex deposits, mesangial cell proliferation and thickening of the capillary wall by mesangial interposition. It causes a minority of cases of childhood and adult nephrotic syndrome. Membranoproliferative GN classically presents as nephrotic syndrome with microscopic hematuria. Occasionally, however, the patient may first come to medical attention because of an acute nephritic picture. About one-half of the patients have low serum C3 and low total hemolytic complement activity levels. The low complement levels have been attributed to the presence in the plasma of C3 nephritic factor, a protein that consumes complement when added to normal serum. The nephrotic syndrome usually persists but may remit leaving persistent proteinuria. End stage renal failure occurs in most of these patients by 10 years after the onset. Opinions differ on whether treatment changes the symptoms or ultimate outcome of this disease. This disease may recur in the transplanted kidney, suggesting the presence of circulating factors, perhaps in this case, circulating immune complexes.

Diagnosis

Nephrotic range proteinuria (more than 3 gm/day) may be discovered during routine urinalysis or during evaluation of edema. Such heavy proteinuria is virtually always caused by glomerular disease with one chief exception. A few patients with **multiple myeloma** may produce massive quantities of antibody light chains (Bence-Jones proteins), which easily pass across the normal glomerular capillary wall because of their low molecular weight. This causes heavy proteinuria without urinary losses of albumin and other plasma proteins. Although the proteinuria might lead one to believe that there is a glomerular disease, urinary protein electrophoresis will show the light chains without any albumin. In 10% of patients with multiple myeloma, however, renal amyloidosis occurs as a complication. In these cases a true nephrotic syndrome may be signalled by hypoalbuminemia, edema and the appearance of albumin in the urine in addition to light chains.

The diagnosis of heavy proteinuria or nephrotic syndrome caused by lupus nephritis, amyloidosis and diabetic glomerulosclerosis is usually suspected from the clinical picture and supported by laboratory studies such as ANA, complement levels, or protein electrophoresis. The presence of amyloidosis may often be confirmed on a biopsy of subcutaneous fat of the abdomen, avoiding the need for a renal biopsy. In patients with lipoid nephrosis, focal sclerosing, membranous and membranoproliferative GN generally one cannot make a diagnosis without a renal biopsy, although a low complement level or gross hematuria would favor membranoproliferative GN. However, in nephrotic children lipoid nephrosis is so common that a renal biopsy is not carried out. Instead, a trial of corticosteroids is given and a good response is taken as evidence for lipoid nephrosis.

Treatment

The ideal treatment for nephrotic syndrome would be to heal the glomerular capillary wall leak. This is only possible in lipoid nephrosis, focal segmental glomerulosclerosis and lupus nephritis, where corticosteroids or cyclophosphamide may be effective after several weeks. Additional methods must be used to control the edema in these diseases before the steroids take their effect or in other diseases that are steroid resistant. These methods are generally aimed at reducing capillary hydrostatic pressure in order to promote reabsorption of edema fluid. One begins by dietary salt restriction. This further reduces extracellular (and intravascular) volume which may already be slightly low due to hypoalbuminemia. If weight loss does not occur, diuretics are employed. When albumin levels are very low, these methods may precipitate symptomatic hypovolemia with orthostatic hypotension or even shock. Intravenous albumin can be used in these extreme cases to restore the blood pressure and promote reabsorption of edema. It is only employed in severe cases, however, since it requires intravenous administration, is expensive and is rapidly lost through the urine.

Chronic Glomerulonephritis

Chronic GN is characterized histologically by a variable amount of sclerosis and proliferation by light microscopy. It is a very common diagnosis at autopsy of patients dying of renal disease or in kidneys from patients with end stage renal disease nephrectomized prior to transplantation. While it may represent an unknown form of GN, it is more likely a common final pathway for the many forms of glomerular disease discussed here. It has been suggested that following renal damage by GN the surviving glomeruli are hypertrophied, hyperperfused and hyperfiltrating in compensation for lost nephrons, and that this hyperfiltration itself produces progressive glomerular damage and sclerosis (see chapter on **renal perfusion disorders**). Clinically, patients who have chronic GN on renal biopsy demonstrate proteinuria, variable numbers of red cells and casts in the urine, usually some impairment of renal function, and occasionally nephrotic syndrome. This disease often goes on to end stage renal disease but may also continue unchanged for many years.

Suggested Readings

Bernard DB. Extrarenal complications of the nephrotic syndrome. Kidney Int 1988; 33:1184–1202.

Cameron JS. The nephrotic syndrome and its complications. Am J Kidney Dis 1987; 10:157–171.

Couser WG. In situ formation of immune complexes and the role of complement activation in glomerulonephritis. Clin Immunol Allergy 1986; 6:267–286.

Glassock RJ. Clinical aspects of glomerular diseases. Am J Kid Dis 1987; 10:181–185.

Glassock RJ. Pathophysiology of acute glomerulonephritis. Hospital Practice 1988; 23:93–108.

Kaysen GA, Myers BD, Couser WG, Rabkin R, Felts JM. Biology of disease, Mechanisms and consequences of proteinuria. Lab Invest 1986; 54:479–498.

Madaio MP, Harrington JT. The diagnosis of acute glomerulonephritis. NEJM 1983; 309:1299–1302.

Mann R, Neilson EG. Pathogenesis and treatment of immune-mediated renal disease. Med Clin North Am 1985; 69:715–750.

Wener MH, Mannik M. Mechanisms of immune deposit formation in renal glomeruli. Springer Semin Immunopathol 1986; 9:219–235.

GLOMERULAR DISEASE PROBLEMS

1. Pick best answer from Column B for each disease in Column A. Each answer may be used once, more than once or not at all.

Column A
1. Polyarteritis nodosa
2. Goodpasture's syndrome
3. Berger's disease
4. Alport's syndrome
5. Acute GN
6. Chronic GN
7. Henoch-Schonlein purpura
8. Idiopathic crescentic GN
9. Nephritis of bacterial endocarditis

Column B
a. Gross hematuria 3 days after sore throat and runny nose
b. Gross hematuria and deafness
c. Gross hematuria and hemoptysis
d. Gross hematuria 15 days after a sore throat
e. Gross hematuria, fever and splenomegaly
f. Gross hematuria, rash and gastroenteritis
g. Gross hematuria, rash and flank pain
h. Found on autopsy after years of proteinuria
i. Blood in the urinary space important in the pathogenesis

2. You are summoned to the emergency room to see a critically ill 10-year-old boy who was diagnosed by his pediatrician as having acute pulmonary edema. The patient has had reduced urine output for one day. An examination shows a blood pressure of 170/130 mm Hg, tachycardia, distended neck veins, gallop rhythm, physical signs of pulmonary edema and generalized edema.

   A. The least likely diagnosis of the following choices is:
   a. Malignant hypertension with congestive heart failure
   b. Congestive heart failure with poor renal perfusion
   c. Poststreptococcal GN
   d. Lipoid nephrosis
   e. Crescentic GN

   B. A more careful examination shows a weeping, crusting skin rash and red cells and red cells casts are noted on urinalysis. The single test more likely to reveal the etiologic agent is:
   a. Cardiac catheterization
   b. Careful retina examination by an ophthalmologist

   c. Skin culture
   d. Anti-GBM antibody test
   e. Creatinine clearance
3. Your patient is referred by a local physician for hypertension, hematuria, proteinuria and increased Scr of unknown duration. After an appropriate evaluation, a renal biopsy is performed. For each of the possible pathological findings in Column A choose the most appropriate answer from Column B. Each answer may be used once, more than once or not at all.

Column A
1. 90% of glomeruli involved by crescents; negative immunofluorescence
2. Diffuse hypercellularity and polys by light microscopy
3. Focal proliferation with diffuse mesangial IgA deposition
4. Focal proliferation with granular IgG and C3 deposition
5. Focal proliferation with linear IF for IgG
6. Unusually thin or layered GBM on EM
7. Variable amount of sclerosis and proliferation

Column B
a. Renal failure progresses over 3 weeks to anuria; patient unlikely to regain much renal function
b. Several siblings with hematuria and hearing aids
c. Hemoptysis may occur in the near future
d. Patient has a rash, arthritis and gastroenteritis
e. Clinical picture likely to slowly worsen or remain unchanged
f. Impetigo; complete recovery likely
g. If patient is febrile, listen carefully for a murmur

4. A 43-year-old nurse has been giving herself weekly booster injections with diphtheria-pertussus-tetanus (DPT) vaccine for 2 years. On a routine urinalysis she is found to have proteinuria and hematuria.
  A. You suspect that she has glomerular injury due to:
    a. Renal allergy to DPT antigens
    b. Chronic exposure to infected patients
    c. Immune complex-mediated GN caused by DPT immune complexes

d. Antibodies to DPT antigens which cross-react to GBM
e. An immune complex GN in which the antigen is unknown, since these make up the majority of cases of immune complex GN.
B. All of the following results would be consistent with this diagnosis EXCEPT:
a. A linear pattern of IF for immunoglobulin
b. Increased BUN
c. Polymorphonuclear infiltrate of glomeruli
d. Glomerular injury noted on renal biopsy
e. Complement deposition in the glomerulus by IF

5. A 40-year-old woman was well until 6 weeks ago when she noted malaise, arthralgias, weight loss, gross hematuria and ankle edema. On physical examination the patient has hypertension, fever (T = 39°), a skin rash, distended neck veins, a third heart sound without a murmur, absent splenomegaly, and a moderate amount of ankle edema. Urinalysis shows blood-tinged urine with 2+ protein, red cells and red cell casts. The Scr is 1.8 mg/dl. The serum C3 and C4 are depressed.
Based on this initial information, the most likely of the following diagnoses is:
a. Polyarteritis nodosa
b. Lupus nephritis
c. Henoch-Schonlein purpura
d. Subacute bacterial endocarditis
e. Alport's syndrome

6. An older patient is admitted with generalized edema. There is a history of diabetes mellitus and both glycosuria and proteinuria on urinalysis.
A. The edema is **least** likely due to:
a. Acute GN in a diabetic
b. Congestive heart failure in a diabetic
c. Diabetic nephropathy with nephrotic syndrome
d. Renal amyloidosis
e. Berger's disease

Your history reveals a recent sore throat, a longstanding draining osteomyelitis of the femur, gradual onset of edema, but no dyspnea on exertion, orthopnea or paroxysmal nocturnal dyspnea.

Your physical exam shows normal blood pressure, normal pulse, normal fundi, flat neck veins, dullness at the bases of the lung fields, no rales, the presence of ascites, no hepatosplenomegaly, 4+ pitting edema up to the umbilicus, and a draining sinus in the right thigh.

B. The **most** likely diagnosis is:
- a. Acute GN in a diabetic
- b. Congestive heart failure in a diabetic
- c. Diabetic nephropathy
- d. Renal amyloidosis
- e. Berger's disease

7. A 23-year-old woman in her 6th month of pregnancy is referred to you because of edema. She has had proteinuria for many years and has developed venous insufficiency of the lower extremities during the pregnancy. In addition, she has mitral insufficiency from childhood rheumatic fever. She denies dyspnea on exertion, orthopnea and paroxysmal nocturnal dyspnea. Her physical examination shows a normal blood pressure and pulse; the neck veins are flat; the murmur of mitral insufficiency is unchanged; the lungs are clear; and the uterus is an appropriate size for her stage of pregnancy. She has varicose veins of the lower extremities, signs of venous stasis and 2–3+ edema. Your laboratory values show: Scr 2 mg/dl, 24-hour urine for protein 5 gm, no hematuria on urinalysis, serum albumin 4 gm/dl (normal 4–5 gm/dl), cholesterol 300 gm/dl (normal 150–230 mg/dl).

The most likely diagnosis is:
- a. Chronic renal disease with edema due to venous stasis
- b. Nephrotic syndrome due to a chronic glomerulopathy
- c. Hypervolemia due to renal insufficiency
- d. Congestive heart failure
- e. Acute glomerulonephritis

8. Pick the best answer in Column B for each item in Column A. Each answer may be used once, more than once, or not at all.

Column A	Column B
1. Focal segmental glomerulosclerosis	a. Has at least three histologic forms
2. Membranous GN	b. Recurs in transplant
3. Renal amyloid	c. May be due to malignancy
4. Diabetic nephropathy	d. Low serum C′ and negative ANA
5. Membranoproliferative GN	e. Increased glomerular perfusion and GBM synthesis
6. Lupus nephritis	f. May complicate chronic inflammation or multiple myeloma
7. Lipoid nephrosis	g. Immunologic disease without immune deposits

9. Select from Column B the most likely cause of nephrotic syndrome (NS) for each patient in Column A:

Column A	Column B
1. A 4-year-old child	a. Focal segmental glomerulosclerosis
2. A young woman with arthritis, fever and rash	b. Membranous GN
3. A 50-year-old man with an acute nephritic picture	c. Renal amyloid
4. A patient with several episodes of steroid-responsive NS who then progresses to chronic renal failure	d. Diabetic nephropathy
5. A young man with peripheral neuropathy and failing vision	e. Membranoproliferative GN
6. A patient with steroid-resistant NS for many years who gradually losses his proteinuria	f. Lupus nephritis
7. A patient with hepatomegaly, a large tongue and low voltage on EKG.	g. Lipoid nephrosis

10. Select from Column B the most likely complication affecting the patients with the nephrotic syndrome in Column A.

Column A
1. A 5-year-old child with a relapse
2. of NS develops fever and abdominal pain
3. An older man with membranous GN develops chest pain on taking a deep breath and coughs up bloody sputum
4. A 40-year-old woman with lupus nephritis and longstanding nephrotic syndrome develops sudden paralysis of the right side of her body
You give diuretics to a patient with renal amyloidosis. He is brought to the emergency room after fainting after getting out of bed

Column B
a. Viral gastroenteritis
b. Pneumonia
c. Myocardial infarction
d. Goodpasture's syndrome
e. Peritonitis
f. Pulmonary embolism
g. Stroke
h. Hypotension
i. Edema of the brain

Table 6.3.
Overview of Glomerular Diseases

Disease	Pathology	Clinical Presentation			Specific Treatment	Prognosis
		Nephritic	Nephrotic	Other		
Diffuse proliferative GN	Diffuse cellularity					
Poststreptococcal GN	PMN's, IC deposits throughout, humps	X		Poststreptococcal infection, ↓ complement	Antibiotics	Most heal
Focal Proliferative GN	Focal segmental cellularity					
Berger's disease	IgA IC in mesangium	X		URI may exacerbate		¼ CRF
Lupus nephritis	IgG IC in mesangium and inside GBM	X	X	Active SLE, ANA+, ↓ complement	Steroids, cyclophosphamide	Most heal
Polyarteritis nodosa	No IC deposits	X		Extrarenal disease	Steroids, cyclophosphamide	⅓ die[a]
Henoch-Schonlein purpura	IgA IC in mesangium	X		Rash, arthritis, gastroenteritis		Most heal
Bacterial endocarditis	IgG IC in mesangium	X		Fever, rash, murmur, ↓ complement	Antibiotics	Most heal
Goodpasture's syndrome	Linear IgG in GBM	X		Pulmonary hemorrhage	Steroids, cyclophosphamide, plasmapheresis	Most CRF

Disease	Morphology / IF	Clinical features			Treatment	Prognosis
Crescentic GN	Crescents in >50% glomeruli		X		Large doses IV steroids	Some heal, some CRF
Idiopathic	Negative, granular (IC), or linear (aGBM AB)IF			X		
All diseases causing focal proliferative GN	(See above)	(See above)			(See above)	(See above)
Alport's syndrome	Thin or layered GBM	Familial hematuria, deafness	X			Men CRF
Amyloidosis	Amyloid fibrils	Extrarenal disease	X			Most die[a]
Diabetic glomerulosclerosis	Widening GBM and mesangium	DM >10 years, retinopathy	X			Most CRF
Lipoid nephrosis	"Fused" foot processes	URI may trigger	Relapsing		Steroids	All heal
Focal segmental glomerulosclerosis	Sclerosed segments in some glomeruli		X		Steroids	¼ respond, ½ CRF
Membranous GN	IC deposits and spikes outside GBM		X			¼ heal, ¼ CRF
Membranoproliferative GN	IC deposits inside GBM, mesangial interposition and ↑ cellularity	↓ complement	X	X		Most CRF

Abbreviations: aGBM AB—antiglomerular basement membrane antibody; ANA—antinuclear antibody; CRF—chronic renal failure; DM—diabetes mellitus; GBM—glomerular basement membrane; GN—glomerulonephritis; IC—immune complexes; IF—immunofluorescence; PMNs—polymorphonuclear leukocytes; SLE—systemic lupus erythematosus.

[a] Death usually caused by extrarenal disease.

chapter 7

Renal Perfusion Disorders

Jaime S. Carvalho

The kidneys regulate the volume and composition of body fluids by forming and then modifying a glomerular filtrate. The process of filtrate formation requires the kidneys to be perfused with an adequate flow of blood at a pressure high enough to overcome the opposing oncotic and hydraulic pressure and the "resistance" to filtration of the glomerular capillary walls. If these perfusion requirements are not met, metabolic waste excretion may be inadequate and renal failure occurs. In contrast, if perfusion increases above normal, irreversible glomerular damage may ultimately result. Before discussing these renal perfusion disorders, it is appropriate to review the blood flow pathways to the glomeruli and the process of filtration.

Normal Renal Circulation and Glomerular Hemodynamics

The renal artery divides successively into segmental, interlobar, arcuate, and interlobular arteries. As they run from the corticomedullary border toward the surface of the kidney, the interlobular arteries give off the afferent arterioles, each supplying one glomerulus (Fig. 7.1). Normally there are no arterioarterial anastomoses between these vessels, which are accordingly functional end arteries. Blood flows through the glomerular capillaries and efferent arterioles into the peri-

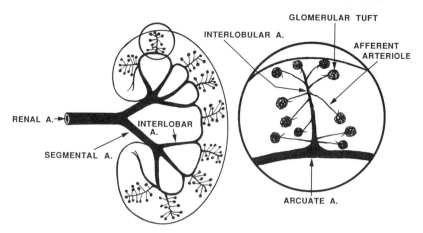

Figure 7.1. Schematic representation of the preglomerular arterial vasculature.

tubular capillaries. Several efferent arterioles from the glomeruli situated at various depths in the cortex supply each tubule. From the peritubular capillaries the blood passes along the interlobular, arcuate, interlobar and segmental veins to finally reach the main renal vein.

With a normal blood perfusion of 3–5 ml/min/gm of tissue, the kidney receives 20% of the cardiac output and is among the most highly perfused organs in the body. Thus, renal cortical blood flow is similar to that observed at maximal vasodilation in myocardium and salivary glands. However, the renal oxygen extraction is low, only 10–15%. This suggests that the high perfusion is not dictated by oxygen need, but rather is a prerequisite for maintaining a high GFR.

The total perfusion of the kidney depends on both the perfusion pressure and the vascular resistance. The diameters of intrarenal arteries, and afferent and efferent arterioles determine the renal vascular resistance and actively change to regulate blood flow.

The blood flow from the renal artery is distributed asymmetrically throughout the renal parenchyma. Approximately 90% of blood traverses just the cortical vessels, approximately 10% also perfuses the outer medulla, and only 1–2% reaches the inner medulla and papilla.

Glomerular hydrostatic pressure depends on arterial blood pressure, so that it is the heart that provides the energy to move fluid across the glomerular membranes. Strictly speaking, the transudation process should be referred to as ultrafiltration. (Filtration implies the separation of gross particulate matter from solution; ultrafiltration implies the separation of gross particulate matter and large colloidal molecules such as proteins from solution, leaving the smaller crystalloid particles such as urea, glucose and salt in solution.) The Starling forces involved in the ultrafiltration process can be represented as:

$$
\begin{aligned}
\text{Net filtration pressure} &= \text{glomerular capillary hydrostatic pressure} \\
&\quad -(\text{capillary colloid osmotic pressure} \\
&\quad + \text{Bowman's space pressure}) \\
&= 60 - (25 + 10) \text{ mm Hg} \\
&= 25 \text{ mm Hg}
\end{aligned}
$$

The GFR is the product of this net filtration pressure, glomerular surface area and glomerular permeability. Since arterial blood pressure is a major factor in net filtration pressure, changes in arterial pressure can cause changes in the GFR. In fact, if the mean arterial pressure were to fall to half its normal value, glomerular filtration would decrease more than proportionately. Such a drop in arterial pressure would reduce the glomerular capillary hydrostatic pressure to such an extent that it would be less than the force attracting fluid into the glomerular capillaries. In this situation glomerular filtration would stop, resulting in complete cessation of renal function. A urinary obstruction that raised capsular pressure by 20–30 mm Hg would also stop glomerular filtration.

Renal Hypoperfusion

Inadequate renal perfusion is a common cause of renal failure and is especially important to diagnose because it is usually treatable if discovered in time.

Etiology

Renal hypoperfusion may be brought about by a variety of disorders and mechanisms, which are listed in Table 7.1. The most common causes of hypoperfusion are the conditions described in Group I: cardiac pump failure, hypovolemia and peripheral vasodilatation. They reduce systemic blood pressure and lead to accumulation of nitrogenous wastes known as prerenal azotemia.

Table 7.1.
Principal Causes of Renal Hypoperfusion

I.   Decreased blood pressure **(prerenal azotemia)**
   A. Primary cardiac pump failure
      1. Acute myocardial infarction
      2. Arrhythmia with low cardiac output
      3. Pericardial tamponade
      4. Any severe cardiomyopathy
   B. Hypovolemia (secondary cardiac pump failure)
      1. Whole blood loss (hemorrhage)
      2. Plasma loss
         a. Renal losses
            i.   Osmotic diuresis, e.g. glycosuria $2°$ diabetes mellitus
            ii. Diuretics
            iii. Aldosterone deficiency, e.g. primary adrenal insufficiency
            iv. Diabetes insipidus
         b. Extrarenal losses
            i.   Gastrointestinal fluid
            ii. Skin losses
            iii. Third spacing
   C. Decrease in systemic vascular resistance
      1. Sepsis
      2. Antihypertensive drugs
II. Renal vascular obstruction
   A. Renal artery embolism
      1. Mural thrombi postmyocardial infarction
      2. Atrial thrombi due to atrial fibrillation
   B. Severe renal artery stenosis or thrombosis
   C. Renal vein thrombosis
III. Altered renal vascular resistance (vasomotor reaction)
   A. Decreased postglomerular resistance
      1. Angiotensin-converting enzyme (ACE) inhibitors
         a. Captopril
         b. Enalapril
   B. Increased preglomerular resistance
      1. Nonsteroidal anti-inflammatory drugs (NSAID)
      2. Hepatorenal syndrome
   C. Unknown mechanism (nephrotoxic reaction to radiocontrast media)

Pathogenesis

To understand the pathogenetic mechanisms involved in the conditions listed in Table 7.1, it is necessary to know how renal blood flow (RBF) and GFR regulation is accomplished in the physiologic state.

Autoregulation

Blood flow in the kidney, as well as that in many other organs, shows **autoregulation**, defined as the intrinsic tendency of an organ to maintain constant blood flow despite changes in arterial perfusion pressure. Thus, in the dog kidney, RBF usually will remain practically constant despite variation in renal arterial pressure from approximately 80–160 mm Hg, i.e. well below and above normal arterial pressure (Fig. 7.2). Appropriate changes in precapillary smooth muscle tone cause the vascular resistance to increase with increasing perfusion pressure, and vice versa. As indicated by the prefix "auto", this is independent of external influences, such as hormones and nerve activity.

The finding that the whole kidney GFR is autoregulated to the same extent as RBF led to the concept that the resistance changes take place only in the preglomerular vessels. However, recent studies have disclosed that variations in arterial pressure may cause changes in efferent arteriolar tone as well. The dominant intrarenal mechanisms that sta-

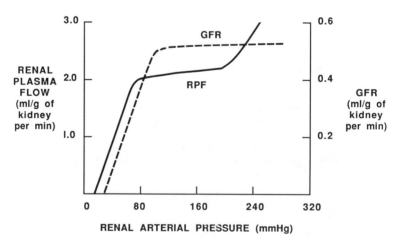

Figure 7.2. Autoregulation of RBF (represented by renal plasma flow—RPF) and GFR.

bilize GFR under normal conditions of pressure and flow are represented in Figure 7.3A.

According to the **myogenic theory,** at normal arterial pressure the preglomerular vessels have a basic myogenic tone, i.e. they are in a state of contraction in the absence of any nervous or humoral stimuli. As arterial pressure falls, the renal vasculature senses arterial pressure changes and decreases myogenic tone. The preglomerular resistance may drop to the level obtained with vasodilator drugs that presumably abolish myogenic tone completely.

Another mechanism involved in the autoregulation of RBF and GFR is known as **tubuloglomerular feedback (TGF).** It is probably located in the macula densa, where it senses flow changes in the distal tubule of each nephron brought about by changes in arterial pressure. An increase in renal perfusion pressure raises GFR, which increases flow rate in the distal tubule of each nephron. This change in flow rate stimulates the TGF mechanism, which causes preglomerular vasoconstriction in that nephron unit. In this way, distal tubular flow returns to normal and in the process, overall GFR and RBF become regulated. These feedback-induced changes in vasomotor tone are caused by a local juxtaglomerular mechanism. However, the nature of the mediator involved and the transmission mechanism from tubular to vascular walls are still unknown. It is believed by some that the TGF mechanism is fast enough and potent enough to explain most, if not all, the GFR autoregulation which occurs with moderate changes in renal arterial pressure.

Other Mediators of Renal Hemodynamics

When renal perfusion pressure is reduced to levels near the lower limits of autoregulation, or when other disturbances such as Na^+ depletion are superimposed on reduced renal arterial pressure, another mechanism comes into play. Increased renin release enhances local formation of angiotensin I. This is converted to **angiotensin II,** which acts locally to increase the *efferent* arteriolar resistance. This raises glomerular capillary hydrostatic pressure and thereby helps to maintain GFR, despite the fact that renal blood flow is reduced (Fig. 7.3B).

Under certain pathophysiologic conditions, the **intrarenal prostaglandins** participate in modulating renal vascular tone. Increased formation of prostaglandins such as *prostaglandin E_2 (PGE$_2$)* leads to renal vasodilation and an excess of *thromboxane A_2 (TXA$_2$)* is associated with renal vasoconstriction. In states of decreased cardiac output

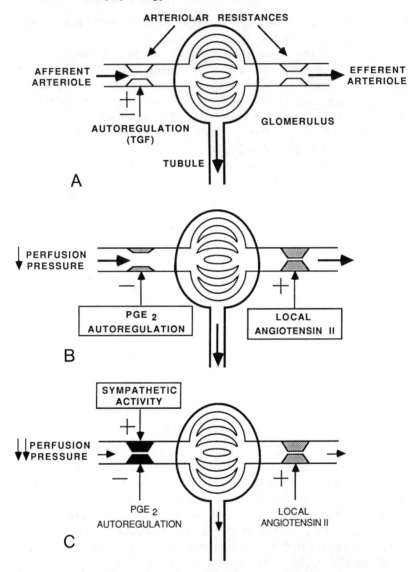

Figure 7.3. Simplified scheme of intrarenal mechanisms for GFR regulation under various hemodynamic conditions. + = vasoconstriction, − = vasodilatation, TGF = tubuloglomerular feedback. A. Normal conditions. B. Perfusion pressure reduced but still within autoregulatory range. C. Prerenal azotemia.

or blood pressure, vasoactive hormones tend to raise preglomerular resistance. However, concomitant increases in renal synthesis of PGE_2 help preserve renal perfusion by reducing this preglomerular vasoconstriction (Fig. 7.3B).

Although inferential data supports a direct correlation between the renal kallikrein-kinin system activity and RBF, no functional role of this system in adjustment of intrarenal vascular resistances has been described.

Prerenal Azotemia

Prerenal azotemia is renal failure brought about by a fall in systemic arterial pressure that impairs renal perfusion. In most cases, **reduced cardiac output** due either to *primary heart disease* or *hypovolemia* decreases blood pressure. Alternatively, **reduced systemic vascular resistance** as seen in septic shock may decrease the blood pressure. Initially, reflex peripheral vasoconstriction in cases with low cardiac output and reflex increase in cardiac output in cases with reduced resistance may minimize the drop in perfusion pressure. However, as the underlying condition worsens, renal perfusion pressure falls.

The normal response of the body to decreased blood pressure includes activation of the sympathetic system and the release of renin and ADH. When renal perfusion pressure starts to diminish, renal autoregulation, angiotensin II and prostaglandins prevent RBF and GFR from falling. However, with marked reduction in perfusion pressure the preglomerular vasoconstriction imposed by the increased sympathetic activity overwhelms these compensatory mechanisms. The resulting reduction in renal blood flow and glomerular capillary hydrostatic pressure will decrease GFR and BUN and Scr will rise (Fig. 7.3C). Less Na^+ is filtered and an increase in isotonic reabsorption of Na^+ takes place in the proximal tubule. Additionally, most of the Na^+ delivered to the distal tubule is reabsorbed by the action of aldosterone, which has been released in response to the high levels of circulating angiotensin II. In the collecting tubule water is rapidly reabsorbed into a hypertonic renal interstitium (maintained by the reduced medullary blood flow) through a collecting tubule wall made highly permeable by the action of ADH. As a result of these tubular actions, a small volume of concentrated urine of high specific gravity and low Na^+ concentration is formed.

If the hypoperfusion is severe enough and sustained for prolonged periods of time acute tubular necrosis may develop (discussed in the chapter on **acute renal failure**).

Renal Vascular Obstruction

Renal Artery Embolism or Thrombosis and Renal Vein Thrombosis. These decrease or completely stop RBF and GFR mainly by mechanical obstruction to blood flow and often result in renal infarction.

Renal Artery Stenosis. During progression of a renal artery stenosis (due to an atherosclerotic plaque or fibromuscular hyperplasia) renal autoregulation initially sustains normal RBF. In addition, when the juxtaglomerular apparatus senses the effects of pressure reduction, the release of renin to the systemic circulation raises the level of circulating angiotensin II. This powerful vasoconstrictor increases arterial pressure, which tends to restore to normal the renal perfusion pressure beyond the stenosis, but may produce severe systemic hypertension (see chapter on **hypertension**). Angiotensin II also increases efferent arteriolar resistance and thereby helps maintain glomerular capillary pressure. RBF and GFR remain constant until the renal artery luminal diameter is reduced by more than 50%. If the high prestenosis perfusion pressure is reduced with antihypertensive drugs, or if progressive stenosis further decreases luminal diameter, a critical poststenotic pressure will be reached and the compensatory ability of autoregulatory dilatation will be surpassed. Glomerular capillary hydrostatic pressure will decrease and GFR will fall below normal.

Altered Renal Vascular Resistance (Vasomotor Reaction)

Angiotensin-Converting Enzyme (ACE) Inhibition. In situations with decreased renal blood flow, GFR depends on angiotensin II-mediated vasoconstriction of the efferent arteriole. Under these conditions, intrarenal blockade of angiotensin II generation reduces glomerular capillary hydrostatic pressure and GFR. Thus, in patients with hypertension due to bilateral renal artery stenosis or to renal artery stenosis of a solitary kidney such as a renal transplant, therapy with an inhibitor of angiotensin converting enzyme, such as captopril or enalapril, may rapidly result in acute renal failure. Often the drug simultaneously reduces blood pressure, but renal failure may occur even if systemic blood pressure is affected little or not at all. (What do you think happens to RBF after captopril?)

Nonsteroidal Anti-Inflammatory Drugs (NSAID). A variety of disease states exist in which administration of a NSAID has major effects on renal function and particularly on GFR. In children with patent ductus arteriosus, administration of indomethacin to effect closure of the ductus is sometimes associated with large decreases in GFR and elevations of Scr. The same can occur when NSAIDs are given to adults who have congestive heart failure or cirrhosis of the liver with prominent ascites. It appears that in these three conditions the cardiac output or effective circulatory volume is reduced and the body responds by activating the vasoconstricting systems, such as the renin-angiotensin and the sympathetic nervous system. Under these circumstances renal prostaglandins such as PGE_2 preserve RBF and GFR by a vasodilatory influence on the afferent arterioles (Fig. 7.3B). When NSAID's are administered, renal prostaglandin synthesis diminishes, resulting in unopposed renal vasoconstriction and increased preglomerular resistance. This reduces glomerular capillary hydrostatic pressure and GFR.

Hepatorenal Syndrome. This is the name given to the unexplained acute renal failure that occurs in patients with severe liver disease usually with ascites. It is due to sustained and marked renal cortical vasoconstriction (particularly of afferent arterioles) which diminishes RBF and GFR. The mediator(s) of this vasoconstriction is unknown. The process is a functional one and reverses with either restoration of liver function (spontaneous or by liver transplantation) or transplantation of the kidneys to a normal environment. With progression of portal hypertension the mesenteric venous vasculature slowly expands its capacity and in addition arteriovenous shunts form within the splanchnic circulation. While total blood volume may increase in this setting the effective arterial blood volume falls, constituting an afferent signal to the renal tubule to augment salt and water retention.

Nephrotoxic Reaction to Radiocontrast Media. Iodine containing contrast media are injected into patients to opacify organs and vessels during angiography, computed tomography and intravenous pyelography. These media may produce a sudden decrease in GFR that usually lasts 3–5 days. The fall in GFR is thought to be due to an acute increase in arteriolar resistance. The exact mechanism is not known.

Clinical Features

Bilateral renal hypoperfusion ultimately leads to a rise in Scr and BUN. The majority of cases are due to prerenal azotemia secondary to one or more of the causes listed in Group I on Table 7.1. Less often a drug, such as captopril or indomethacin (a NSAID), is responsible for the hypoperfusion, but even in these cases, an abnormally low systemic blood pressure can be a predisposing factor. It is imperative, therefore, to evaluate the volume and hemodynamic status of any azotemic patient.

The history and physical examination often will reveal or suggest the cause of renal hypoperfusion, e.g. fever, chills and hypotension in septic shock. Hypovolemic patients may complain of severe thirst or lightheadedness on standing. They may have jugular veins that do not fill with the patient lying flat, tenting of the skin or dryness of the oral mucous membrane. If hypovolemia is suspected, blood pressure and pulse rate should be checked for orthostatic changes in recumbency and 3–5 minutes after the upright position is assumed. Normally, systolic and diastolic pressure drop less than 15 mm Hg and pulse rises less than 15 beats/minute when a person assumes the upright posture.

In cases of unilateral renal vascular obstruction, the rise in Scr and BUN is attenuated by the continuing function of the contralateral kidney. Renal artery embolism often produces abdominal, flank or back pain. Patients with azotemia caused by renal artery stenosis will usually have hypertension that has been increasingly difficult to control. Auscultation of the abdomen or costovertebral angles may reveal a bruit transmitted from the stenotic renal arteries.

Diagnosis

Prerenal azotemia can usually be recognized thanks to the appropriate physiological responses of stimulation of aldosterone and other mediators of renal Na^+ retention. They enhance tubular reabsorption of Na^+ and typically reduce the urine Na^+ concentration to less than 20 mEq/L. Similarly, reduced effective blood volume in hepatorenal syndrome, reduced blood pressure due to ACE inhibitors and reduced renal Na^+ excretion in patients on NSAID often reduce urine Na^+ concentration below this level.

In cases of decreased systemic blood pressure or decreased "effective" circulating volume ADH is also released. Thus in prerenal azotemia and hepatorenal syndrome urine-specific gravity and urine osmolality are frequently high (specific gravity > 1.020, Uosm > 350 mOsm/kg). Urine volume is usually under 500 ml/day when azotemia develops. In prerenal azotemia the reduced urine flow is accompanied by increased tubular reabsorption of urea and the BUN/Scr ratio is usually greater than 20:1.

If one is unsure of vascular volume, it can be more directly assessed by measuring right atrial pressure with a central venous catheter and/ or left atrial pressure (pulmonary capillary wedge pressure) with a Swan-Ganz catheter. This catheter also allows measurement of cardiac output, using a thermodilution modification of the Fick principle. If there is still a question of inadequate renal blood flow, a trial of volume expansion with intravenous saline or albumin solution may be undertaken to see if GFR improves.

High peripheral vein renin levels may be found in patients with renal artery stenosis severe enough to cause azotemia. Radioisotope scanning will show reduced or absent perfusion of one or both kidneys in case of renal embolism.

Treatment

The treatment is directed at the specific cause of the renal hypoperfusion. When volume depletion is at fault, the volume must be replaced with appropriate fluid (see chapter on **volume disorders**). If a diuretic drug is responsible for hypovolemia it should be discontinued, as should an antihypertensive vasodilator drug that produces hypotension beyond the autoregulatory range of the renal vasculature. When inhibitors of angiotensin-converting enzyme or prostaglandin synthesis are responsible for the renal dysfunction, GFR usually improves after the offending drug is discontinued. Renal artery stenosis may be corrected by surgical repair or by percutaneous transluminal balloon dilation. The latter is accomplished by way of a catheter introduced percutaneously into a femoral artery and directed under fluoroscopic guidance into the stenotic region of the renal artery. The stenosis is then dilated by inflating a balloon near the tip of the catheter.

Renal Hyperperfusion

Under some circumstances, the glomeruli may have chronically increased blood flow and filtration rates. It has been hypothesized that this hemodynamic state may cause progressive glomerular damage in various clinical situations.

Etiology

Several of the known causes of glomerular hyperperfusion are listed on Table 7.2.

Table 7.2.
Principal Causes of Glomerular Hyperperfusion

I. With normal nephron mass
   A. Early diabetic glomerulosclerosis
   B. Sickle cell anemia
   C. Pregnancy
   D. High protein intake
II. With diminished nephron mass
   A. Solitary kidney
      1. Congenital
      2. Nephrectomy
   B. Nephron loss by disease, e.g. poststreptococcal GN

Pathogenesis

It has been known for years that in the early stages of juvenile onset diabetes mellitus, RBF and GFR are higher than normal. The cause of these changes is not clear, but may involve expansion of extracellular volume, increased glomerular prostaglandin production and reduced preglomerular arteriolar resistance. This observation led to the hypothesis that increased glomerular pressures and blood flows and the resultant hyperfiltration could produce the glomerular damage (diabetic glomerulosclerosis) that causes proteinuria, and, ultimately, renal failure. According to the **hyperfiltration hypothesis,** these hemodynamic alterations are capable of inducing endothelial and epithelial cell damage, which increases glomerular permeability to albumin and leads to albuminuria. The increased leakage of albumin overburdens and damages mesangial cells. As a result, there is proliferation of mesangial cells and increased formation of mesangial matrix, which ultimately leads to the glomerular sclerosis.

Theoretically, the harmful effect of glomerular hyperfiltration could occur whenever RBF and GFR are elevated, as in sickle cell anemia, pregnancy and high protein intake. The glomerulosclerosis occasionally seen in longstanding sickle cell anemia could be an example of this. There are no proven deleterious renal effects of pregnancy or high protein intake, but it is conceivable that the protein-rich diet of Western society contributes to the glomerulosclerosis "normally" seen with aging.

Similar hemodynamic factors may be responsible for the manifestations of glomerular damage seen in some patients with single functioning kidneys. The nephron population of such individuals is reduced to half, but through poorly understood compensatory mechanisms, these remaining nephrons undergo hypertrophy and increase their glomerular capillary pressure, blood flow and **single nephron GFR.** The high single nephron GFR brings total renal GFR back toward or to the normal range. While most individuals with solitary kidneys suffer no adverse effects, some develop mild proteinuria and a very rare patient has nephrotic syndrome and progressive renal failure associated with glomerulosclerosis. It is hypothesized that hyperfiltration may cause the glomeruli in solitary kidneys to sclerose and further reductions in the number of nephron units impose ever increasing hemodynamic stresses on the remnant nephrons, eventually leading them to irreversible failure.

This deleterious long-term effect of high single nephron GFR in compensation for lost nephrons could explain why diverse forms of human renal disease, such as poststreptococcal GN, do not always display stable renal insufficiency after the original insult is removed and immunologic damage ceases, but occasionally manifest worsening chronic renal failure. Indeed, this mechanism has been proposed to play a role in the progression of chronic GN and, in fact, of all diseases with slowly deteriorating renal function.

So far, most of the studies supporting the above hypothesis have been done in rats. For instance, rats with nephrectomy of ⅚ of renal tissue or diabetes mellitus have high single nephron GRF and develop proteinuria and worsening renal insufficiency associated with progressive glomerulosclerosis. A protein restricted diet in these rats reduces single nephron GFR and halts or slows down the rate of progression of the renal damage. Similar beneficial results have also been obtained by treatment of these rats with an ACE inhibitor to prevent systemic hypertension and glomerular hyperfiltration from developing. Whether hyperfiltration can induce structural damage in human kidneys still remains to be demonstrated. Also, as of this date no adequately designed controlled study is available to demonstrate beyond doubt the efficacy of protein restriction or of ACE inhibitors in retarding the progress of chronic renal disease in man.

Suggested Readings

Badr KF, Ichikawa I. Prerenal failure: A deleterious shift from renal compensation to decompensation. NEJM 1988; 319:623–629.

Bank N, Klose R, Aynedjian HS, Nguyen D, Sablay LB. Evidence against increased glomerular pressure initiating diabetic nephropathy. Kidney Int 1987;31:848–905.

Brenner MG, Meyer TW, Hostetter TH. Dietary protein intake and the progressive nature of kidney disease: the role of hemodynamically mediated glomerular injury in the pathogenesis of progressive glomerular sclerosis in aging, renal ablation and intrinsic renal disease. N Engl J Med 1982;307:652–659.
Ferguson RK et al. Clinical applications of angiotensin-converting enzyme inhibitors. Am J Med 1984;77:690–698.
Lifschitz MD. Renal effects of nonsteroidal anti-inflammatory agents. J Lab Clin Med 1983;102:313–323.
Ofstad J, Aukland K. Renal circulation. In: Seldin W and Giebisch G, eds. The kidney. New York: Raven Press, 1985:471–496.
Papper S. Hepatorenal syndrome. Contrib Nephrol 1980;23:55–74.

RENAL PERFUSION DISORDER PROBLEMS

1. A 57-year-old housewife is known to have an invasive squamous cell carcinoma of the oropharynx and normal kidney function. She was brought to the emergency ward for inability to swallow food and weight loss of several weeks' duration. She was cachectic and had dry mucous membranes and markedly decreased skin turgor. The systolic blood pressure was 80 mm Hg; the temperature was 97°F; and the respiratory rate 22/minute. The mouth showed a fungating mass involving most of the oropharynx, but the remainder of the physical exam was unremarkable. Initial laboratory studies revealed a BUN of 58 mg/dl and a Scr of 2.2 mg/dl. Which **one** of the following urinary findings is most likely to be found in this patient:

	Urine Na$^+$ concentration (mEq/L)	Urine osmolality (mOsm/ kg)	Urine flow rate (ml/hour)
a.	65	1014	3
b.	8	286	10
c.	3	908	15
d.	42	810	21
e.	13	860	50

2. A 58-year-old man with longstanding hypertension and severe peripheral vascular disease on a diuretic was found to have blood pressure of 190/110 mm Hg. At the time BUN was 25 and Scr 1.5 mg/dl. Captopril was then added to the therapeutic regime. Three

weeks later he feels well; BP is 145/85 mm Hg with no significant postural changes, but BUN is found to be 40 and Scr 3.8 mg/dl. Which **two** of the following statements are true?

a. His cardiac output has been drastically reduced.
b. His impairment of kidney function may be related to the drop in arterial pressure.
c. The patient is unlikely to recover the lost kidney function.
d. Bilateral renal artery stenosis may be present.
e. Captopril may have produced vasomotor changes that increased renal vascular resistance.

3. The conditions in Column A have altered renal hemodynamics resulting in abnormal GFR. Match each condition with the most appropriate description of renal hemodynamic status from Column B.

Column A

1. Primary adrenal insufficiency
2. Bilateral renal artery stenosis
3. New onset diabetes mellitus
4. Hepatorenal syndrome

Column B

	Perfusion pressure	Preglomerular arteriolar resistance	Plasma flow	GFR
a.	↓	↓	↓	↓
b.	Normal	↓	↑	↑
c.	Normal	↑↑	↓	↓
d.	↓	↑	↓	↓

4. In a patient with new onset diabetes mellitus, which two of the following therapeutic maneuvers might theoretically help prevent glomerular damage?

a. Immunosuppressive therapy with corticosteroids
b. Low protein diet
c. Administration of an ACE inhibitor
d. Maintenance of normal blood glucose concentration with diet and drugs

5. A 59-year-old woman was admitted for elective cardioversion. She had several months' history of idiopathic chronic atrial fibrillation, but no other symptoms. Her blood pressure was 140/90 mm Hg and the pulse was 90/min and irregular. On the day after cardio-

version, she was in normal sinus rhythm when she suddenly experienced severe left flank pain associated with nausea and vomiting. The Scr rose from 1 to 1.9 mg/dl. Which **one** of the following statements is more likely to be true?

  a. She should be treated with large spectrum antibiotics until urine culture results are available.
  b. The pain in the left flank is most likely unrelated to the left kidney.
  c. A radioisotope renal scan will probably show differences in blood flow to the kidneys.
  d. An intravenous pyelography should demonstrate a filling defect in the left ureter.

6. A 49-year-old chronic alcoholic was admitted to the hospital with mild jaundice, ascites and peripheral edema. Blood pressure was 135/85 mm Hg. The BUN was 8 and Scr 0.9 mg/dl. Urine Na^+ concentration was 32 mEq/L. He was treated with bed rest, low Na^+ diet and diuretics. The liver disease worsened. After 2 weeks of treatment, body weight increased and blood pressure was unchanged but he became oliguric. BUN rose to 40 mg/dl and Scr rose to 3.5 mg/dl. Pulmonary capillary wedge pressure was normal. Plasma osmolality was 285 and urine osmolality 625 mOsm/kg. Urine Na^+ concentration measured on 3 consecutive days showed the following values: 12, 8 and 3 mEq/L. Which **one** of the following statements is true?

  a. Azotemia is due to a fall in plasma volume from the Na^+ restricted diet and diuretics.
  b. Azotemia is unrelated to the decline in liver function.
  c. Azotemia is due to high peripheral vascular resistance.
  d. Azotemia is due to high renal vascular resistance.
  e. Azotemia is the result of high colloid osmotic pressure in glomerular capillaries.

7. GFR is maintained in the face of falling blood pressure by all of the following **EXCEPT**:
  a. Increased local generation of angiotensin II
  b. Increased renal sympathetic activity
  c. Increased renal synthesis of PGE_2
  d. Suppression of tubuloglomerular feedback
  e. Decreased preglomerular myogenic vascular tone

chapter 8

Disorders of Urinary Outflow

Sewell I. Kahn

Obstructive Uropathy

Obstruction of the urinary flow is a common cause of renal failure. It is important to make the diagnosis since early recognition and treatment can often restore renal function.

Definitions

Obstructive uropathy is defined as changes in the urinary system due to an obstruction to urinary outflow. Dilatation of the collecting system in the kidney is called **hydronephrosis** and changes in kidney function are called **obstructive nephropathy.**

There are multiple methods of classification of obstruction. Obstruction may be complete or partial, unilateral or bilateral and acute or chronic. Obstruction may occur at a number of sites in the urinary tract including the tubules and collecting ducts (renal), and the renal pelvis, ureter, or urethra (postrenal).

Etiology

The causes of urinary obstruction are numerous, therefore, only the most common conditions will be listed (Table 8.1).

Pathogenesis

Mechanisms of Urine Outflow Obstruction

There are many ways by which urine flow may be blocked. First, **intrinsic renal** obstruction can occur in multiple myeloma when immunoglobulin light chains are filtered and then precipitate in the tubules. Second, **postrenal** obstruction can arise through an *internal* blockage of the collecting system. For example, urinary stones can form in the kidney and then move into and obstruct the ureter, or a carcinoma of the bladder can grow into and close off the vesical outlet. Third, obstruction due to *external* compression on the system may be caused by a tumor of a contiguous organ, e.g. carcinoma of the cervix, or a nonmalignant disease such as an enlarged prostate, retroperitoneal fibrosis or a pregnant uterus. Although pregnancy frequently causes hydronephrosis, it rarely impairs renal function or produces clinically significant obstruction. Finally, a neurogenic bladder may not empty and cause a functional obstruction.

Table 8.1.
Principal Causes of Obstructive Uropathy

I.   Renal, e.g. myeloma proteins
II. Postrenal
    A. Urinary stones
    B. Benign prostatic hypertrophy
    C. Congenital ureteropelvic or ureterovesical obstruction
    D. Tumors
        1. Prostate
        2. Bladder
        3. Cervix or ovary
        4. Colon
    E. Retroperitoneal fibrosis
    F. Neurogenic bladder dysfunction
        1. Spinal cord trauma
        2. Neurologic disease, e.g. multiple sclerosis, diabetic neuropathy

Renal Blood Flow and Glomerular Filtration

Obstruction of the urinary outflow of the kidney causes changes in renal blood flow, glomerular filtration and tubular function. Most studies have been done on experimental animals and the findings extrapolated to man.

The renal hemodynamic response to obstruction is in three phases (Fig. 8.1): 1) Initially a decrease in afferent arteriolar resistance, perhaps involving vasodilating prostaglandins, results in a rise in renal blood flow. This is associated with an increased intraureteral pressure. 2) After 2–5 hours of obstruction, renal blood flow declines but intraureteral pressure continues to rise. An increased afferent arteriolar resistance mediated by thromboxane or the renin-angiotensin system is responsible for this fall in renal blood flow. 3) Finally, possibly due to low urinary flow, intraureteral pressure declines toward or to normal levels.

A fall in GFR is caused initially by increased Bowman's space pressure and later by reduced blood flow and capillary hydrostatic pressure.

There is some residual glomerular filtration in both partial and complete obstruction. In complete obstruction, the filtered salt and water is reabsorbed by the tubules and returned to the lymphatics. GFR may be markedly decreased in an obstructed kidney and obstruction of a solitary kidney or bilateral obstruction can cause severe renal failure.

Tubular Function

During Partial Obstruction. The partially obstructed kidney often loses distal tubule functions, such as the ability to concentrate the urine and the ability to excrete an acid load, leading to nephrogenic diabetes insipidus and distal RTA.

After Relief of Obstruction. Renal function following release of obstruction deserves some comment. In experimental animals, after short-term complete obstruction (less than 30 hours) both the GFR and renal blood flow return to normal. In long-term obstruction only minimal recovery of glomerular filtration is observed.

Bilateral obstruction can also grossly impair tubular function following release of obstruction. Urinary loss of salt and water may be large. This **postobstructive diuresis** is caused by: 1) volume overload, which occurs during bilateral obstruction, 2) accumulation of poorly reabsorbed solutes, such as urea, that act as osmotic diuretics, 3) intrinsic

NORMAL

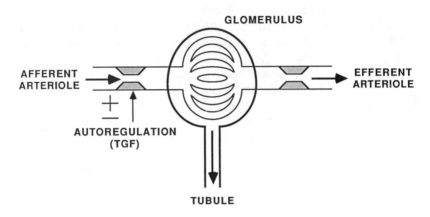

OBSTRUCTION (PHASE 2)

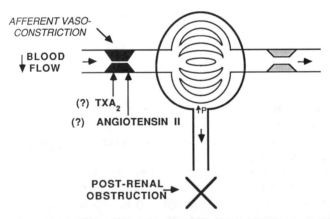

Figure 8.1. Schematic representation of mechanisms that reduce GFR in obstruction. In phase 1 increased renal blood flow and capillary hydraulic pressure partially offset the rise in Bowman's space pressure. In phase 2 vasoconstriction reduces capillary hydrostatic pressure and further compromises GFR. In phase 3 low urine flow allows Bowman's space pressure to fall, but continued vasoconstriction maintains low GFR.

OBSTRUCTION   (PHASE 1)

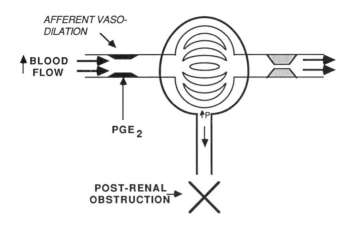

*AFFERENT VASO-
DILATION*

↑ BLOOD
FLOW

PGE$_2$

POST-RENAL
OBSTRUCTION

OBSTRUCTION   (PHASE 3)

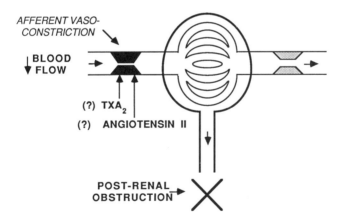

*AFFERENT VASO-
CONSTRICTION*

↓ BLOOD
FLOW

(?) TXA$_2$

(?) ANGIOTENSIN II

POST-RENAL
OBSTRUCTION

tubular defects or a retained hormonal agent, which decrease tubular reabsorption of Na^+, probably at the thick ascending limb of the loop of Henle, and 4) unresponsiveness to ADH. The latter may be due to depletion of the solute content of the papillary interstitium secondary to increased relative blood flow in papillary structures or due to unresponsiveness to ADH of the tubular cells themselves reflected by a decrease in cyclic AMP production.

An **acidifying defect** is also seen in the postobstructed kidney. This may be due to decreased H^+ production or problems in the reabsorption of HCO_3^-.

Clinical Features

The major manifestations of urinary tract obstruction are pain, changes in urine flow and a decrease in renal function. Pain may vary from absent to severe. The passage of a stone through a ureter causes the most intense pain, renal colic, and is discussed below in the section on **renal calculi.** Partial obstruction may cause polyuria, while complete obstruction bilaterally or obstruction to a solitary kidney may cause anuria. Obstruction of bladder outflow as seen with benign prostatic hypertrophy can lead to dribbling, a weak urinary stream, straining to achieve bladder emptying and hesitancy, i.e. delay in starting the urinary stream while bladder pressure builds to overcome the resistance.

We shall see in the chapter on **acute renal failure** that obstruction or **postrenal azotemia** is one of the three principal mechanisms that cause azotemia. Therefore, obstructive uropathy must be considered as a cause of renal failure of unknown etiology.

Diagnosis

The diagnostic approach should include history, physical examination, laboratory and radiologic procedures and clinical maneuvers.

It is important to get information regarding urinary output (anuria or polyuria), difficult or abnormal micturition, flank, abdominal or suprapubic pain and drug usage. (Anticholinergic medications may impair bladder function.) Physical examination should be done looking for a flank or suprapubic mass or tenderness. Rectal examination in men may reveal prostatic hypertrophy or carcinoma, while pelvic examination in women can show a gynecologic malignancy. A urinalysis is important since hematuria and crystaluria suggest kidney stones. Urinary tract infections may complicate obstruction and result in white cells and bacteria in the urine. There is usually no proteinuria with obstructive lesions.

If severe flank pain suggests renal stone disease, the approach should be a plain X-ray of the abdomen to see radiopaque stones and an intravenous pyelogram (IVP). IVPs involve the intravenous injection of a contrast agent, i.e. an organic compound that is iodinated to make it radiopaque. When the compound appears in the collecting system after filtration by the glomeruli and concentration by the tubules, an X-ray of the abdomen shows some opacification of the parenchyma and marked opacification of the calyces, pelvis and lower urinary tract. Urinary obstruction produces dilatation of the collecting system that is easily seen (Fig. 8.2).

If abnormal micturition suggests obstruction at the level of the bladder outlet, one should insert a Foley catheter right after the patient has voided and measure the urine remaining in the bladder. A **residual urine volume** of >100 cc would be evidence of inadequate bladder emptying due to neurogenic bladder dysfunction or bladder outlet obstruction, as seen with benign prostatic hypertrophy.

If flank pain or unexplained renal failure raises the question of obstruction above the bladder, one should proceed with either an IVP or a renal ultrasound. Ultrasonography produces an image of the kidneys by sending high frequency sound waves into the body and recording waves reflected off internal structures. Ultrasonography detects dilatation of the calyces in almost all cases of obstruction but has a number of false positives (Fig. 8.3). An IVP provides more accurate information than an ultrasound, but may itself cause renal failure in older patients and may not show the collecting system at all in severe renal failure. If further delineation of urinary tract lesions is needed, retrograde pyelograms may be performed by passing a cystoscope through the urethra and by using the cytoscope to insert catheters up the ureters. A contrast agent is then injected up the catheters. Retrograde pyelograms are rarely needed to diagnose obstruction, but they are useful to localize and characterize the obstructing lesion. Computer-assisted tomographic (CAT) scans are useful to define anatomically underlying causes of obstruction such as tumor, retroperitoneal fibrosis, etc.

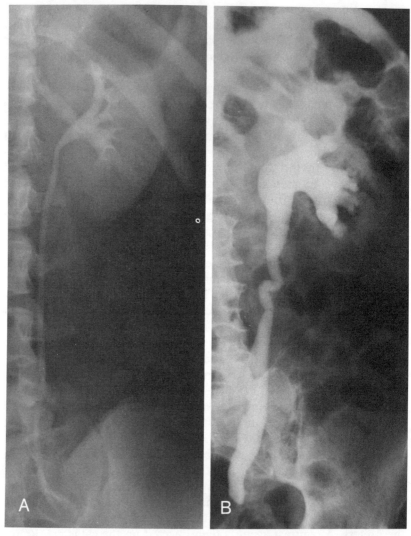

Figure 8.2. (A) Normal IVP. (B) IVP showing hydronephrosis and hydroureter.

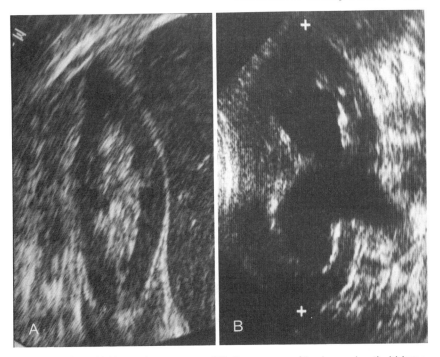

Figure 8.3. (A) Normal sonogram. (B) Sonogram of hydronephrotic kidney showing dilated calyces.

Treatment

The primary treatment for obstruction is to relieve it. Unilateral stones up to 1 cm in diameter often pass spontaneously. Obstruction below the bladder is treated temporarily with a urethral catheter. Working through a cystoscope, the urologist may place a retrograde ureteral catheter or stint past an obstruction of the ureter. In certain circumstances, an antegrade catheter may be placed percutaneously into the kidney to temporarily drain the urine and relieve the obstruction. If possible, the underlying cause i.e. tumor, stone, etc. should be treated.

Relief of obstruction of a few days' duration generally results in return of GFR to normal. Relief of obstruction of weeks' or months' duration should be attempted, as partial recovery of GFR may be observed.

Renal Calculi

Renal stones occasionally produce renal failure due to obstruction and may rarely even lead to chronic renal failure. Their main clinical importance, however, is as a cause of pain and morbidity in stone formers, who are responsible for 1 in 1,000 hospital admissions.

Etiology

Renal calculi form by precipitation of a substance from urine that is oversaturated with that substance. Stones may be composed of any of several chemical species and may occur in a variety of conditions (Table 8.2).

Pathogenesis

Physical Chemistry of Stone Formation

In order to understand the pathogenesis of stones, one must understand the activities of crystals in solutions (Fig. 8.4). The tendency for a solute to precipitate from solution depends on the **activity product** of

Table 8.2.
Principal Causes of Renal Calculi

I.   Calcium stones
    A. Hypercalciuria
        1. Idiopathic
        2. Hyperparathyroidism
        3. Distal renal tubular acidosis
        4. Sarcoidosis
    B. Uricosuria
    C. Hyperoxaluria
    D. Idiopathic (normocalciuric)
II. Uric acid stones
    A. Overproduction
        1. Gout
        2. Hematologic malignancies
    B. Persistently acid urine
        1. Idiopathic
        2. Chronic diarrhea
III. Magnesium ammonium phosphate stones (infection with urea splitting bacteria)
IV. Cystine stones (cystinuria)

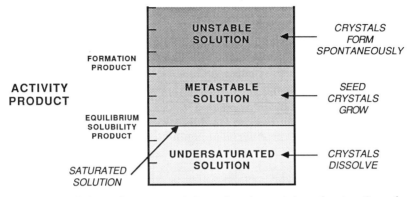

Figure 8.4 Schematic representation of various states of saturation of a substance in solution.

the free ions in that solution (e.g. for calcium oxalate: $[Ca^{2+}] \times [oxalate^-]$).

Undersaturated Solution. In an undersaturated solution added crystals will dissolve. The activity product is less than the **equilibrium solubility product.**

Saturated Solution. In a saturated solution crystals, e.g. calcium oxalate, will not change in size, i.e. they are in equilibrium with the solution. Addition of more free ions (e.g. Ca^{2+} and/or oxalate$^-$ to a solution of calcium oxalate) would cause the crystals to grow. Removal of ions would cause the crystals to shrink. The activity product of a saturated solution equals the equilibrium solubility product.

Metastable Solution. A metastable solution contains free ions in a concentration above the saturation level, but no crystal formation appears. However, if crystals were already present or if seed crystals were added to the solution they would grow.

Unstable Solution. An unstable solution is more concentrated than a metastable one and has a free ion concentration so high that spontaneous crystal formation occurs. The activity product that marks transition from a metastable to an unstable state is known as the **formation product.**

These definitions and conditions should tell us something about stone formation:

1) If the activity product of calcium oxalate in the urine is in the metastable range, i.e. more than saturated, and crystals are present in the urine, they will grow. If a crystal of another species is present, there

may also be growth on that species. For example, calcium oxalate crystals may form on a crystal of uric acid. This is called **heterogeneous nucleation.** It should be noted that the activities of solutes are often in the metastable range in **normal** urine! The absence of preformed crystals may prevent stone formation in normal individuals. Alternatively, microscopic crystals may be washed away before they grow large enough to be caught in the kidney.

2) If the activity product of the solute is in the unstable range, i.e. above the formation product, then spontaneous stone formation will occur. Thus the factors that raise the concentration of ions should favor stone formation. Either **increased crystalloid excretion,** e.g. hypercalciuria, hyperuricosuria etc., or **decreased water excretion** due to low water intake or high insensible losses will increase stone formation. **Changes in pH** can markedly effect the activity of ions in solution and therefore contribute to the formation of stones. **Inhibitors** are substances in the urine which bind free ions (such as Ca^{2+} or oxalate$^-$) and form soluble complexes. These substances therefore decrease the activity product and decrease the formation of stones. Urine contains a number of inhibitors, such as pyrophosphates, acid mucopolysaccarides, citrates and magnesium ion. Many inhibitors are specific for certain types of stones.

In a given population, there are those who have a tendency to form stones and those who do not form stones. The majority of stone formers, but not all, have recognizable metabolic abnormalities. Conversely, many people with these same metabolic abnormalities do not form stones, suggesting that other factors, such as absence of inhibitors, play a role in stone formation.

As mentioned above, renal calculi may be composed of a variety of substances. Table 8.3 shows the composition of stones in a population of stone formers and reveals that most stones are made up of Ca^{2+}, usually as the oxalate salt.

Calcium Stone Disease

A population of patients with Ca^{2+} stones may be further subdivided according to metabolic abnormality (Table 8.4).

Only the most common causes of Ca^{2+} stones will be discussed.

Hypercalciuria. The amount of Ca^{2+} in the urine varies somewhat with net intestinal absorption. The upper limit of normal for Ca^{2+} excretion on a normal diet is 300 mg/24 hours in the male and 250 mg/24 hours in the female. Patients who excrete more than this are

Table 8.3.
Types and Prevalences of Renal Stones[a]

	% Prevalence	
Type	Adults	Children
Calcium oxalate	32.7	
Calcium phosphate	3.4	
Calcium oxalate and phosphate	34.3	57
Magnesium ammonium phosphate with calcium oxalate or phosphate	19.0	31
Uric acid	5.8	5
Cystine	2.9	5

[a] Data taken from EL Prien. J Urology 61:821, 1947 and MS Polinski, BA Kaiser, HJ Baluarte. Urolithiasis in childhood. Pediatr Clin NA 34:683, 1987.

labelled **hypercalciuric.** Hypercalciuria may be due to increased bone resorption (e.g. hyperparathyroidism), decreased renal tubular reabsorption of Ca^{2+} (e.g. distal renal tubular acidosis), or increased gastrointestinal absorption of Ca^{2+} (e.g. sarcoidosis). If all known causes of hypercalciuria are excluded the patient is said to have idiopathic hypercalciuria.

Table 8.4.
Prevalences of Underlying Disorders in Calcium Stone Formers[a]

Type	Prevalence (%)
Hypercalciuria	43.3
Idiopathic	32.2
Hyperparathyroidism	5.2
RTA	3.7
Sarcoidosis	0.7
Medullary sponge kidney	1.5
Hyperuricosuria	14.6
Hypercalciuria and hyperuricosuria	11.7
Hyperuricemia	5.7
Secondary hyperoxaluria	4.6
No metabolic disorder	20.2

Data from FL Coe. Nephrolithiasis. Pathogenesis and treatment. Chicago: Yearbook Medical Publishers, Inc. 1978:6.

Idiopathic hypercalciuria accounts for approximately 40% of all calcium oxalate stone disease. It is usually found in middle age men and there is often a strong family history of urolithiasis. There are two major types of idiopathic hypercalciuria: (1) *intestinal hyperabsorption* of Ca^{2+} and (2) *renal tubular leak* of Ca^{2+}.

Hyperparathyroidism causes approximately 5% of Ca^{2+} stone disease. These stones tend to be of calcium phosphate (hydroxyapatite) or calcium oxalate. Hyperparathyroidism may also cause nephrocalcinosis, i.e. calcification of the renal parenchyma. One sees both increased Ca^{2+} and phosphate in the urine because parathormone increases resorption of bone, increases activation of vitamin D (and consequently intestinal Ca^{2+} and phosphate absorption) and reduces tubular reabsorption of phosphate.

Distal RTA is associated with calcium phosphate stones and nephrocalcinosis. Distal RTA is characterized by systemic acidosis and a relatively alkaline urine. The buffering of H^+ by the bone in the chronic acidemic state causes resorption of bone and release of Ca^{2+} and phophorus. In addition, acidosis decreases renal tubular reabsorption of Ca^{2+} and decreases citrate (an inhibitor) in the urine. The elevated pH in the urine plays a major role by decreasing the solubility of calcium phosphate.

Normocalciuria. Some individuals form Ca^{2+} stones despite normal urinary Ca^{2+} excretion.

Hyperuricosuria is found in approximately 25% of patients with calcium oxalate stones and a few have hyperuricemia. The cause of this relationship is not clear, however, there is evidence that the uric acid crystals have lattice dimensions, which allow for crystal growth by heterogenous nucleation in a metastable calcium oxalate solution. In addition, the uric acid may absorb inhibitors in the urine so favoring calcium oxalate precipitation.

Hyperoxaluria is a rare cause of stone disease. Oxalate is an end product of metabolism and is also present in the diet. *Hereditary biochemical defects* may increase oxalate production, while *gastrointestinal diseases* can result in excessive oxalate absorption from the gut.

No metabolic abnormality is found in the idiopathic group of Ca^{2+} stone formers. It is possible that these patients are missing some inhibitor in the urine.

Uric Acid Stones

Uric acid stones make up approximately 5% of all stones in the adult. The formation of uric acid stones is favored by 1) an increase in uric acid excretion usually above 800 mg/24 hours, 2) a decrease in urine volume and most importantly, 3) an acid urine. Overproduction of uric acid accounts for the increase in uric acid stone formation in gout. Also, lymphoproliferative and myeloproliferative diseases, especially when treated, cause a marked increase in uric acid production.

One of the most common causes of uric acid stones is not overproduction of uric acid, but deficient ammonia production. This leads to a constantly acid urine, which promotes the precipitation of uric acid by favoring the conversion of soluble urate to relatively insoluble uric acid: $H^+ + Na^+$ urate$^-$ (soluble)$\rightarrow Na^+$ + uric acid (insoluble).

Chronic diarrheal states, such as inflammatory bowel disease, favor uric acid stone formation, since the loss of water and bicarbonate in the stool lead to the production of a concentrated acidic urine.

Magnesium Ammonium Phosphate Stones

These are the so-called infection or struvite stones, which occur in the face of urinary tract infections with urea-splitting organisms, usually Proteus species. The urease produced by these bacteria generates ammonia and carbonate from urea in the urine. The increase in pH from ammonia favors the precipitation of magnesium ammonium phosphate often with Ca^{2+} carbonate apatite (Ca_{10} ($PO_4)_6 \cdot CO_3$). This combination of magnesium, ammonium and calcium phosphate leads to the term "triple phosphate stones."

Cystinuria

Cystinuria causes cystine stones and is due to an inherited metabolic defect in the proximal renal tubular reabsorption of filtered cystine, along with arginine, lysine and ornithine.

Clinical Features

Stone formation is primarily a disease of young and middle adulthood. Only 1% of all stones occur in patients under the age of 10 years.

When stones are in the pelvis or calyces they are usually clinically silent and are often found incidently on X-rays performed for other reasons. Stones that suddenly block the ureter or ureteropelvic junction usually present with pain. The pain associated with renal stone disease may vary, but it is typically that of **renal colic** characterized by severe cramping. It usually begins in the costovertebral angle or flank on the affected side and radiates forward and downward toward the groin, characteristically into the labia in females or into the testis in males. Occasionally, only a part of the pain may be present, such as the pain only in the flank region, or suprapubic area. Renal colic is typically a violent pain, which is anxiety producing and unrelieved by positioning. Consequently, the patient may be restless, constantly moving and occasionally assuming varying postures, such as being doubled up with the knees drawn up to the chest. The pain may last only a few minutes, but characteristically remains for hours to days until the stone passes into the bladder. It may be accompanied by nausea and vomiting and often a paralytic ileus. Because of this, it can be confused with intraabdominal problems. During the attack, the patient may have dysuria and frequency. Although renal colic is the most common type of pain associated with renal stone disease, the pain can be less dramatic with patients complaining of a constant dull ache.

Objective signs may be limited to flank or abdominal tenderness. Paralytic ileus, however, may produce decreased bowel sounds. Patients passing a stone usually have either macroscopic or microscopic hematuria. Complications of renal stone disease include **obstruction** of urinary flow and progressive damage with **permanent loss of function** of the kidney. If the contralateral kidney has been previously damaged or removed, **acute renal failure** will ensue. Approximately 50% of the patients with renal stones have **urinary infections** or even **bacteremia,** and, therefore, signs of infection such as pyuria, leukocytosis and high fevers with accompanying renal colic can be the presenting symptoms of stone disease.

Following passage of a stone most, but not all, individuals will have a recurrence within 5–10 years and many of these will go on to form further stones during their lifetime.

Infection stones tend to be staghorn calculi, i.e. they enlarge to fill and take on the staghorn form of the pelvis and calyces and are difficult to treat (Fig. 8.5). They may lead to intermittent sepsis and hematuria and often result in loss of kidney function.

Diagnosis

The presence of a renal calculus is usually suggested by renal colic. It is occasionally discovered in the investigation of acute renal failure or hematuria or accidentally on a plain X-ray of the abdomen. Most renal stones, with the exception of uric acid stones, contain Ca^{2+} or sulfur, are radiopaque, and may be seen with a plain X-ray of the abdo-

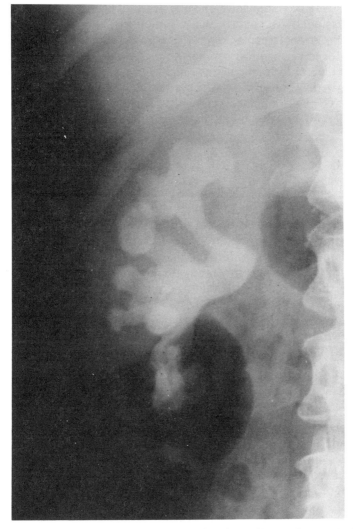

Figure 8.5 Plain X-ray of the abdomen of patient with staghorn calculus.

men. An IVP or sonogram must be done to visualize a uric acid stone or occasionally to confirm that a radiopacity is really in the urinary tract. Stones obtained at surgery or passed spontaneously can be analyzed for their chemical composition. One may wish to look for metabolic defects in frequent stone formers by analyzing a 24-hour urine for Ca^{2+}, oxalate, uric acid or cystine. Patients with infection stones will have an ammoniacal odor to their urine, a positive urine culture (usually proteus) and a very high urine pH (8–9).

Treatment

The pain of renal colic is treated with narcotics. A high fluid intake will produce a diuresis to help advance the stone through the ureter. In general, large stones do not obstruct the ureteropelvic junction or enter the ureter and remain asymptomatic. Small stones (<0.5 to 1 cm. diameter) will pass through the ureter over hours to days. Stones that produce hydronephrosis and do not move after a few days require active therapy, such as basketing from below through a cystoscope, surgical removal or ultrasonic disruption (directly by application of an ultrasonic probe through a percutaneous transrenal approach or indirectly with extracorporeal shock wave lithotripsy).

Prevention

Increased water intake should reduce the urinary concentration of whatever solute(s) are involved. Prevention of further stone formation depends on the underlying disease. Calcium excretion in idiopathic hypercalciuric or even idiopathic normocalciuric Ca^{2+} stone formers may be reduced with thiazides. Patients with hyperparathyroidism can undergo parathyroidectomy. Citrate may be given as an inhibitor of calcification in Ca^{2+} stone disease. In cases with hyperuricosuria, the reduction of uric acid production with diet or allopurinol may decrease further formation of calcium oxalate or uric acid stones. Oral $NaHCO_3$ may further inhibit uric acid stone formation by alkalinizing the urine and in patients with Ca^{2+} stones due to RTA may correct systemic acidemia. In patients with magnesium ammonium phosphate stones, a urease inhibitor, acetohydroxamic acid, decreases ammonia production and may prevent or even dissolve the staghorn calculi.

Suggested Readings

Bordier P, Ryckewart A, Gueris J, Rasmussen H. On the pathogenesis of so-called idiopathic hypercalciuria. Am J Med 1977;63:398.

Broadus AE, Thier SO. Metabolic basis of renal stone disease. NEJM 1979;300:839.

Coe FL, Fauus MJ. Disorders of stone formation. Chapter 32. In: Brenner BM and Rector FC, eds. The kidney. Philadelphia: WB Saunders, 1986:1403.

Klahr S, Buerkert J, Morrison A. Urinary tract obstruction. Chapter 33. In: Brenner BM and Rector FC, eds. The kidney. Philadelphia: WB Saunders, 1986:1443.

Wilson DR. Urinary tract obstruction. Chapter IV. In: Schrier RW and Gottschalk CW, eds. Diseases of the kidney. Boston: Little, Brown and Company, 1988:715–746.

Smith LH. Urolithiasis. Chapter IV. In: Schrier RW and Gottschalk CW, eds. Diseases of the kidney. Boston: Little, Brown and Company, 1988:785–814.

DISORDERS OF URINARY OUTFLOW PROBLEMS

1. Obstruction of the urinary system may cause:
   a. Anuria
   b. Oliguria
   c. Polyuria
   d. No change in the amount of urine
   e. All of the above
2. Obstruction of the urinary system:
   a. May be relieved without regard to duration of obstruction since the blood flow in the obstructed kidney does not change and no long-term damage is done
   b. Must be relieved quickly because the longer the duration of obstruction, the more damage is done to the kidney
   c. Should not be relieved if obstructed for more than 24 hours because irreversible damage has already occurred
   d. Should be treated by removing the kidney since the obstructed kidney can act as a source for infection
3. The renal hemodynamic response to urinary tract obstruction is:
   a. An initial decrease in renal blood flow followed by an increase in renal blood flow
   b. An initial decrease in renal blood flow with no later rise
   c. An initial increase in renal blood flow with no later decrease
   d. An initial increase in renal blood flow followed by a decrease in renal blood flow

4. Postobstructive diuresis is caused by:
   a. Excretion of solutes retained during the period of obstruction
   b. Volume overload
   c. Defects in tubular function
   d. Unresponsiveness of renal tubules to ADH
   e. All of the above
5. Which of the following statements about the use of ultrasonography to diagnose urinary tract obstruction is true?
   a. Ultrasonography will only detect major obstruction of the urinary tract
   b. Ultrasonography will detect almost all cases of obstruction of the urinary tract
   c. When ultrasonography shows obstruction, other tests will always confirm that the urinary tract is obstructed
   d. Since ultrasonography can occasionally cause renal failure when used to diagnose obstruction of the urinary tract, an intravenous pyelogram should always be done first
6. A metastable solution is:
   a. A solution in equilibrium with crystals
   b. A solution in which there is no spontaneous crystal formation, but if seed crystals were added they would grow
   c. A solution in which there is spontaneous crystal formation
   d. A solution with an activity product less than the equilibrium solubility product
   e. A solution with an activity product more than the formation product
7. The most common stones are:
   a. Uric acid stones
   b. Calcium stones
   c. Magnesium ammonium phosphate stones
   d. Cystine stones
   e. Oxalate stones
8. All of the following of the underlying abnormalities has been associated with stone formation **EXCEPT:**
   a. Hypercitricosuria
   b. Sarcoidosis
   c. Hyperparathyroidism
   d. Hyperuricosuria
   e. Hypercalciuria

9. Which of the following are symptoms seen in stone disease?
    a. Clinically silent
    b. Renal colic
    c. Hematuria
    d. Dull aching flank pain
    e. All of the above
10. "Infection stones" are:
    a. Composed of calcium oxalate
    b. Composed of uric acid
    c. Found in patients with persistently alkaline urine
    d. Found in patients with persistently acid urine
    e. Any stones complicated by urinary infections

chapter 9

Acute Renal Failure

Thasia G. Woodworth

Acute renal failure is a common, potentially serious, clinical syndrome occurring in about 5% of patients hospitalized at major medical centers. It may be an isolated problem due to a primary renal disease, but usually is caused by disorders of other organ systems. Although most individuals with mild-to-moderate renal failure are asymptomatic, those progressing to severe renal failure suffer the unpleasant symptoms of uremia and may die of the complications, if the correct diagnosis is not made and appropriate treatment given.

Definitions

Acute renal failure is the sudden inability of the kidneys to regulate salt and water balance appropriately and to clear metabolic wastes, the latter leading to accumulation of nitrogenous breakdown products. Clinicians measure the serum concentrations of two of these products, urea and creatinine, to gauge the severity of the renal failure. Renal failure also leads to accumulation of other substances, such as phosphorus, K^+ and uric acid and to abnormal regulation of body osmolality, volume and acid-base status. Most patients with acute renal failure have an abrupt decline in urine output to <500 cc daily called **oliguria.** Other patients with decreased clearance of nitrogenous wastes continue to excrete 1–2 L of urine daily and are said to have **nonoliguric acute renal failure.**

Etiology

About 70% of patients with acute renal failure have acute tubular necrosis, but many other causes are recognized (Table 9.1).

Pathogenesis

Acute renal failure may be seen with structurally normal tissue in pre- and postrenal azotemia or may result from intrinsic renal disease.

Prerenal Azotemia

Prerenal azotemia is due to decreased blood pressure, with consequent reduced perfusion of normal kidneys. A moderate fall in renal artery perfusion pressure may be counteracted initially by dilatation of the preglomerular arterioles and constriction of the postglomerular arterioles. However, if blood pressure falls below the range of autoregulation (below about 60 mm Hg systolic blood pressure), GFR will fall. In older individuals, and patients with underlying renal disease, less severe falls in blood pressure even to the low normal range, may lead to prerenal azotemia.

Postrenal Azotemia

The other type of acute azotemia with structurally normal renal tissue is called **postrenal azotemia** and is due to obstructive uropathy. As discussed in the chapter on **disorders of urinary outflow,** it can occur with intrinsic obstruction of the collecting system by stones or tissue, or with extrinsic compression by tumors or retroperitoneal fibrosis.

Intrinsic Renal Failure

Renal failure may be seen in a wide variety of primary renal diseases. It may also occur in extrarenal or multisystem diseases, such as polyarteritis nodosa, when there is secondary renal involvement. Generally, in each condition damage to one of the four main parts of the kidney accounts for loss of function of the involved nephrons. For example:

Vascular Disease. The renal blood vessels may become mechanically obstructed by emboli, stenosis or thrombosis or may undergo

Table 9.1.
Principal Causes of Acute Renal Failure

I. Prerenal Azotemia
   A. Primary cardiac pump failure
      1. Acute myocardial infarction
      2. Arrhythmias with low cardiac output
      3. Pericardial tamponade
      4. Any severe cardiomyopathy
   B. Hypovolemia
      1. Whole blood loss (hemorrhage)
      2. Plasma loss
         a. Renal losses
            i.   Osmotic diuresis, e.g. glycosuria 2° diabetes mellitus
            ii. Diuretics
            iii. Aldosterone deficiency, e.g. primary adrenal insufficiency
            iv. Diabetes insipidus
         b. Extrarenal losses
            i.   Gastrointestinal fluid
            ii. Skin losses
            iii. Third spacing
   C. Decreased systemic vascular resistance
      1. Sepsis
      2. Antihypertensive medications
II. Postrenal Azotemia
   A. Urinary stones
   B. Benign prostatic hypertrophy
   C. Congenital ureteropelvic or ureterovesical obstruction
   D. Tumors
      1. Prostate
      2. Bladder
      3. Cervix or ovary
      4. Colon
   E. Retroperitoneal fibrosis
   F. Neurogenic bladder dysfunction
      1. Spinal cord trauma
      2. Neurologic disease, e.g. multiple sclerosis, diabetic neuropathy
III. Intrinsic Renal Failure
   A. Vascular disease
      1. Renal vascular obstruction
         a. Renal artery embolism
         b. Bilateral renal artery stenosis or thrombosis
         c. Renal vein thrombosis
      2. Altered renal vascular resistance
         a. Decreased postglomerular resistance (ACE inhibitors)
         b. Increased preglomerular resistance (NSAID, hepatorenal syndrome)
         c. Unknown mechanism (nephrotoxic reaction to radiocontrast media)

Table 9.1.
Principal Causes of Acute Renal Failure (*Continued*)

  B. Glomerular disease (any nephritic disease)
  C. Tubular disease
      1. Acute tubular necrosis
         a. Ischemia
         b. Toxins, e.g. aminoglycoside antibiotics, myoglobin
      2. Tubular obstruction by myeloma proteins
  D. Interstitial disease (acute interstitial nephritis)
      1. Allergic reaction to drugs, e.g. penicillin analogs or diuretics
      2. Idiopathic

---

changes in resistance. This leads to a fall in blood flow or glomerular capillary hydrostatic pressure and subsequent reduction in GFR.

Glomerular Disease. The glomeruli may be so altered in crescentic or acute glomerulonephritis that reduced permeability and filtering surface severely affect GFR.

Tubular Disease. The tubules may be obstructed in multiple myeloma by immunoglobulin light chains. This has been called myeloma kidney or cast nephropathy.

More commonly the tubules in acute tubular necrosis *(ATN)* undergo ischemic or toxic damage which, together with disturbances of glomerular filtration, impairs renal function. From what we now know, it is clear that ATN results from a complex and poorly understood disease process and much more investigation needs to be done to elucidate its pathogenesis.

In ATN **tubular** injury affects renal function by two mechanisms: 1) *Tubular obstruction* by cellular debris increases Bowman's space pressure, thereby reducing GFR, and 2) *backleak of filtrate* from damaged tubules dissipates tubular fluid. In addition, **arteriolar** and **glomerular** injury affect renal function by a third and fourth mechanism in ATN. The renal insult may 3) *decrease glomerular blood flow* directly through arteriolar necrosis, and glomerular endothelial cell swelling or indirectly through reflex vasoconstriction and mediators like angiotensin II or thromboxane. Similarly, the renal insult may 4) *decrease intrinsic glomerular ultrafiltration capacity* through mediators or direct cell injury which reduce permeability and surface areas of the glomerular capillaries (Fig. 9.1). From animal experiments we know that the relative influence of each of these four mechanisms depends on the nature of the insult, e.g. ischemia, aminoglycoside, etc.

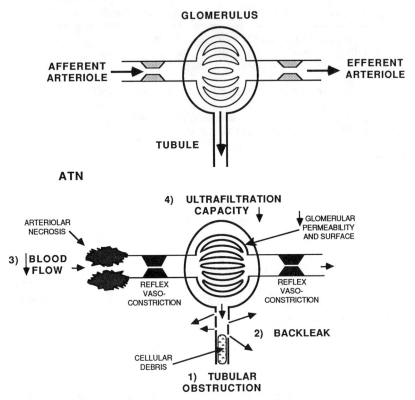

Figure 9.1. Schematic representation of the four pathogenic mechanisms in ATN.

Interstitial Disease. The renal interstitium may be the site of a vigorous inflammatory reaction in allergic interstitial nephritis secondary to drugs. The immunological mechanism is not known. GFR decreases, possibly through secondary damage to the tubules or extrinsic pressure on the tubules by interstitial edema.

Clinical Features

The first manifestation of acute renal failure is a rise in BUN and Scr, accompanied in many cases by a decrease (**oliguria**) or complete cessation of urine output (**anuria**). Patients often have only minor symptoms until the Scr rises above 8–10 mg/dl. Then, several clinical manifestations of acute renal failure may be observed, including hypervolemia, hyperkalemia, metabolic acidosis, hyponatremia and **uremic** symptoms, such as anorexia and vomiting (discussed in the next chapter on **chronic renal failure**). Other clinical features depend on the etiology of the renal failure:

Prerenal Azotemia

This condition results from reduced blood pressure that may come about in three general ways: 1) **Primary cardiac disease**—most commonly due to myocardial infarction with low cardiac output. 2) **Volume depletion**—most commonly due to excess diuretics, bleeding or gastrointestinal fluid losses. 3) **Reduced peripheral vascular resistance**—most commonly due to sepsis. Physical signs of cardiac pump failure or hypovolemia, such as diaphoresis, pallor and confusion are often present.

Postrenal Azotemia

In postrenal azotemia patients often experience a sensation of generalized back fullness or achiness, or acute flank pain, the severity being greater the more rapidly obstruction has occurred. With prostatic or bladder outlet obstruction other complaints may include straining on urination, weak urinary stream, sensation of incomplete bladder emptying, or dribbling. Pelvic neoplasms or prostatic enlargement may be found on rectal or pelvic examination.

Intrinsic Renal Failure

Vascular Disease. A vasomotor reaction may occur due to severe liver disease or the use of NSAID's, radiocontrast media or ACE inhibitors like captopril (see chapter on **renal perfusion disorders**). Alternatively patients with atrial fibrillation or a recent myocardial infarction may have renal emboli, which commonly cause abdominal, back or flank pain. When bilateral renal artery stenosis produces azotemia, months of worsening hypertension may have been observed (see chapter on **hypertension**).

Glomerular Disease. Acute glomerulonephritis may be seen 1–4 weeks after a streptococcal pharyngitis or skin infection. A rash, fever or arthritis raises the possibility of glomerular involvement due to bacterial endocarditis, vasculitis or collagen vascular disease. Tea-colored gross hematuria is highly suggestive of an acute nephritic disease.

Tubular Disease. Myeloma patients typically have anemia and bone pain. However, tubular disease is far more commonly due to ischemic or nephrotoxic **ATN,** the major single cause of all cases of acute renal failure. ATN usually follows hypotension or shock, exposure to a nephrotoxic antibiotic or massive release of myoglobin from muscle injured by ischemia, trauma, etc. A fall in urine output occurs in a majority of patients, but some will continue to excrete 1–2 L of urine daily (nonoliguric ATN), in spite of a decrease in excretion of nitrogenous wastes. Nonoliguric ATN patients have a better prognosis and appear to recover more quickly. The clinical course of ATN includes an **initiation phase,** lasting minutes to days in which the reduction in GFR will reverse with correction of hypotension; the **maintenance phase,** usually lasting 2–4 weeks, in which the GFR remains depressed despite removal of the insult; and the **diuretic phase,** during which almost complete recovery occurs over one to several weeks.

Interstitial Disease. Patients with acute **(allergic)** interstitial nephritis often have fever, rash or eosinophilia and are receiving a penicillin analog, diuretic or other drug known to produce this problem.

Prognosis

The prognosis of acute renal failure reflects the seriously ill condition of the type of patient who usually develops ATN. These individuals are typically old, have multiple diseases and often are critically ill. As a result, despite introduction of dialysis and modern intensive care techniques, the 50% mortality observed in patients in the 1950s, continues to be reported. Infectious complications, gastrointestinal bleeding and other underlying diseases are still the major cause of morbidity and mortality.

Diagnosis

Acute renal failure usually comes to medical attention through an elevated BUN or Scr. Rising Scr levels will usually distinguish acute from chronic renal failure, where levels tend to be stable.

In most cases, the cause of acute renal failure will be suspected or evident from the history and physical examination. Common examples would be the patient with ATN revealed by a history of oliguria following several hours in shock or the elderly man with obstruction from benign prostatic hypertrophy revealed by a history of increasing difficulty in voiding.

Important laboratory tests include Scr, BUN, urine Na^+ concentration and urinalysis including specific gravity, and microscopic examination (Table 9.2). Such urine tests should be performed prior to the administration of diuretics, which affect specific gravity and Na^+ concentration of urine.

The tubules generally function well in prerenal azotemia, acute glomerulonephritis and renal failure associated with altered vascular resistance. They continue to remove Na^+ efficiently from a reduced amount of filtrate, usually resulting in a low urine Na^+ concentration (<20 mEq/L). High ADH levels in prerenal azotemia and hepatorenal syndrome typically produce a concentrated urine. This enhanced water reabsorption slows urine flow in the tubule, allowing increased reabsorption of urea and leading to a BUN:Scr ratio $>20:1$. In contrast, due to loss of tubular function urine Na^+ concentration in postrenal azotemia and ATN is generally high (>40 mEq/L) and urine concentration is isotonic with plasma (specific gravity ~ 1.010; ~ 300 mOsm/kg).

Patients with obstruction by tumors or stones may have hematuria and those with obstruction complicated by infection may have pyuria. Patients with acute nephritic diseases have proteinuria, hematuria and often red cells casts. In ATN urinalysis typically discloses "muddy brown" granular casts and some proteinuria ($\leq 2+$). In allergic interstitial nephritis, white cells appear in the urine sediment occasionally with many eosinophils.

Other laboratory tests that may be of value in assessing the patient with acute renal failure are serologic tests characterizing the various forms of glomerulonephritis: serum complement components and anti-streptolysin O, antihyaluronidase, anti-DNAse, antinuclear and anti-GBM antibodies. For the diagnosis of multiple myeloma, urine and serum protein electrophoreses are obtained. Selection of such tests depends on the clinical setting, of course.

Ultrasonic examination of the renal parenchyma and collecting system may reveal dilatation of the renal pelvis and calyces due to urinary obstruction. It should be done in any undiagnosed case of acute renal failure, since symptoms of obstruction may not always be present. The renal ultrasound may also show small renal size and typical parenchymal changes in cases with chronic irreversible kidney disease.

Table 9.2.
Typical Urinary Findings in Various Forms of Acute Renal Failure

Type of Azotemia	U volume <500 cc/day	Specific Gravity	U_{Na} (mEq/L)	Proteinuria	Urine Sediment
Prerenal	+	>1.020	<20	0	Negative
Postrenal	Variable	~1.010	<20 early <40 late	0	Red or white cells
Altered vascular resistance	Variable	~1.010[a]	<20	0	Negative
GN	Variable	~1.010	<20	2–4+	Red cells, red cell casts
ATN					
(Oliguric)	+	~1.010	>40	0–2+	"Muddy brown" casts
(Nonoliguric)	–	~1.010	>40	0–2+	"Muddy brown" casts
AIN[b]	Variable	~1.010	variable	0–3+	White cells, often eosinophils

[a] >1.020 in hepatorenal syndrome.
[b] AIN—allergic interstitial nephritis.

Treatment

Simultaneous evaluation and treatment are often necessary when acute renal failure is first noted. Detection and correction of hypotension and hypovolemia are important to prevent progression of prerenal azotemia to established ATN. For example repletion of intravascular volume often leads to a rapid rise in urine output and improvement in azotemia. If oliguria is still present after correcting hypovolemia and hypotension, one becomes concerned about **hypervolemia,** since large volumes of fluid may be administered to provide nutrition and medications. The diuretic furosemide may be given to increase urine output. If a diuresis does not occur, ideally one should restrict fluid and Na^+ intake to insensible (sweat, respiratory) losses, plus urine and gastrointestinal output, although this may not be feasible.

All potentially nephrotoxic drugs, such as aminoglycosides, ACE inhibitors and NSAID should be discontinued, if possible. Dosages of renally excreted drugs must be modified. Many pharmacy resource manuals, including the PDR *(Physicians' Desk Reference),* contain information for dosage changes in renal failure.

Potassium balance is often affected. Reduced urinary K^+ excretion particularly with oliguria, and increased tissue breakdown with severe illness can result in K^+ accumulation. Hyperkalemia ($K^+ > 6.5$ mEq/L) is immediately life-threatening, and therefore, serum K^+ must be monitored at least daily. The treatment of hyperkalemia is covered in the chapter on **potassium disorders.**

Acidosis develops slowly, reflected by a progressive fall in plasma HCO_3^- concentration. Bicarbonate administration will be required only in the severely catabolic patient who produces large amounts of acid.

Attention should be given to providing necessary calories and essential amino acids through nutritional support to the catabolic patient who is unable to eat. However, in the oliguric patient the large amounts of fluid used to administer adequate nutrition may cause hypervolemia.

When acute renal failure is severe (GFR <10 ml/min) and lasts for more than a few days, dialysis may be necessary to clear metabolic wastes, remove fluid including that given with nutrition and drugs, and restore electrolyte homeostasis. The two types of dialysis, hemo- and peritoneal, will be discussed in the next chapter on **chronic renal**

failure. The absolute indications for dialysis in acute renal failure include:

1) Severe hypervolemia
2) Hyperkalemia not controlled by conservative means
3) Severe acidosis (HCO_3^- < 10 mEq/L)
4) Uremic symptoms (BUN > 100 mg/dl)

Prevention

Prevention of acute renal failure is the best management. This includes identification of patients at risk, attention to fluid balance, monitoring of BUN and Scr, and careful use of aminoglycosides, ACE inhibitors, potent diuretics, NSAID, and radiocontrast media. The presence of risk factors such as advanced age, hypovolemia, septic shock, diabetes mellitus, congestive heart failure and preexisting chronic renal failure should alert the physician to exercise additional care in management of such patients.

Suggested Readings

Arbeit LA, Weinstein SW. Acute tubular necrosis. Med Clin North Am 1981;65:147–163.
Cronin RE. The patient with acute azotemia. In: Schrier RW, ed. Manual of nephrology. Boston: Little, Brown & Company, 1985;135–150.
Epstein FH, Brown RS. Acute renal failure: Collection of paradoxes. Hosp Pract 1988;23:157–180.
Goldstein MB. Acute renal failure. Med Clin North Am 1983;67:1325–1341.
Hou SH, Buchinsky DA, Wish JB, Cohen JJ, Harrington JT. Hospital-acquired renal insufficiency: A prospective study. Am J Med 1983;74:243–248.
Schrier RW. Acute renal failure: pathogenesis, diagnosis, and management. Hosp Pract 1981;101–112.

ACUTE RENAL FAILURE PROBLEMS

Six cases representing various kinds of acute renal failure are described. After the case descriptions are various possible physical findings, urinalysis and laboratory results, clinical courses and diagnoses. Pick the one answer in each category which best fits each case. Each answer should be used once.

Case 1: A 62-year-old Polish window cleaner presented to his family physician having developed progressive fatigue, loss of appetite and difficulty sleeping over a 1-week period. He had also noted progressive decline in his urine output for the same period, along with a backache. He found this decline in urine output strange, since previously he had noted frequency of urination and nocturia 4–6 times nightly. He denied dysuria or change in urine color. His only medication was diazepam for insomnia.

The family doctor noted a pulse of 86/min, blood pressure of 160/80 mm Hg, bilateral flank tenderness and suprapubic tenderness. Laboratory data disclosed a BUN of 140 mg/dl, Scr of 6.5 mg/dl, Hgb 14.2 g/dl and electrolyte concentrations (mEq/L) of Na^+ 135, K^+ 5.8, HCO_3^- 18 and Cl^- 102.

The patient is then referred to you for further evaluation and management.

Case 2: A 71-year-old man presented to the emergency room with a chief complaint of crampy abdominal pain, nausea of several days' duration and recent onset of vomiting of foul-smelling material. He had 3 years previously undergone abdominal-perineal resection for rectal carcinoma and had a colostomy. The patient took propranolol 40 mg b.i.d. for hypertension.

Physical examination disclosed blood pressure 130/70 mm Hg, temperature 98.6°F, pulse 90/min and regular. Abdomen was distended with hyperactive bowel sounds. The colostomy drained liquid brown stool.

The patient was admitted for further evaluation. X-rays of the abdomen disclosed dilated loops of small bowel with air-fluid levels. Urine output is 10–15 cc/hr. BUN was 110 mg/dl, Scr 3.1 mg/dl and you are called for further diagnostic input.

Case 3: A 34-year-old white male presented to the outpatient clinic with a 5-day history of "cold symptoms" and a 1-day history of shortness of breath, severe cough, chills, high fever, vomiting and decreasing urine output. Past medical history is negative.

Physical examination disclosed a confused, toxic-appearing man. Temperature was 105°F, respiratory rate 30/min, pulse 120/min and blood pressure 100/50 mm Hg. Lungs showed diffuse inspiratory and expiratory rhonchi and there was no audible heart murmur. There was no edema.

Chest X-ray showed a patchy pneumonia with abscess formation. Shortly after admission, blood pressure was noted to be 80/50 mm Hg and IV normal saline was administered and Foley catheter was placed. Broad spectrum antibiotic treatment with a cephalosporin and aminoglycoside was given. BUN was 24 mg/dl and Scr 1.2 mg/dl.

Twenty-four hours later, the patient was still hypotensive and urine output was 10–15 cc/hr. BUN was 32 mg/dl and Scr was 2.9 mg/dl. You are called to aid in further evaluation and management. Despite normalization of blood pressure, there is no change in urine output and Scr continues to rise.

Case 4: A previously healthy 74-year-old white female with no history of diabetes, hypertension or urinary tract problems was hospitalized. She had failed to respond to ampicillin treatment of a bronchitis.

Symptoms included a dry cough, lethargy, itching and nausea. Physical exam disclosed a blood pressure 150/80 mm Hg, pulse 90/min and regular, temperature 100.8°F and normal respirations. Scr is found to be 5.5 mg/dl with a BUN of 50 mg/dl. You are called in consultation.

Case 5: A 42-year-old female with a 5-year history of intermittent fever, leukopenia and polyarthralgia presented to her physician with a 1-week history of dark urine, progressive ankle edema and an exacerbation of arthralgias. She had also noted fatigue, loss of appetite and periorbital edema on arising in the morning. The doctor found a weight increase of 10 lbs, blood pressure 160/110 mm Hg, and 3+ ankle edema. BUN was 90 mg/dl and Scr 8 mg/dl. The patient is referred to you for further evaluation.

Case 6: A 68-year-old man with a previous history of myocardial infarction and recently exacerbated hypertension visited his cardiologist for routine evaluation. Blood pressure was 160/100 mm Hg, so enalapril (5 mg daily) was added to his antihypertensive regimen. Two weeks later, he returned for follow-up. Blood pressure was still 160/100 mm Hg and laboratory evaluation disclosed a serum K^+ concentration of 6.0 mEq/L and a rise in BUN from 18 to 50 mg/dl and Scr from 1.5 to 3.5 mg/dl. The patient is referred for further evaluation.

Physical Findings:

a. Somnolence, fine macular rash and excoriations from scratching
b. Standing blood pressure 160/90 mm Hg, abdominal bruit, weak pulses of the lower extremities
c. Pericardial friction rub, bladder palpable just below umbilicus, prostate firm, walnut-sized, trace pretibial edema
d. Malar rash, pericardial friction rub
e. Standing blood pressure 100/60 mm Hg, pulse 120/min, dry mucous membranes, no edema

f. Blood pressure 180/100 mm Hg, abscess formation over sternum, sacral and thigh edema

Urinalyses:

a. SG[a] 1.012, 1+ protein, pigmented and granular casts, tubular epithelial cells
b. SG 1.030, negative glucose and protein, occasional granular cast, occasional hyaline cast
c. SG 1.015, 1+ protein, granular and WBC casts, 10–20 WBC/hpf with eosinophils
d. SG 1.020, negative protein, occasional hyaline casts
e. SG 1.009, negative glucose and protein, microscopic hematuria, occasional WBC
f. SG 1.015, 4+ protein, microscopic hematuria, RBC casts

Further Laboratory Studies:

a. Urine Na^+ 40 mEq/L, ultrasound: dilated calyces and ureters
b. Urine Na^+ 19 mEq/L, ultrasound: normal-sized kidneys, fluorescent antinuclear antibody 1:640, renal biopsy: widespread immune complex deposits, diffuse proliferation of cells in glomeruli
c. Urine Na^+ 5 mEq/L, ultrasound: normal-sized kidneys
d. Urine Na^+ 18 mEq/L, ultrasound: small right kidney, borderline-sized left kidneys. Renal angiogram: atherosclerotic plaques at both renal artery orifices
e. Urine Na^+ 40 mEq/L, ultrasound: normal-sized kidneys, WBC and differential count: 10% eosinophilia, renal biopsy: normal glomeruli, inflammatory cells in interstitium
f. Urine Na^+ 60 mEq/L, blood cultures: + Staphylococcus aureus, ultrasound: normal-sized kidneys

Clinical Course:

a. Foley catheter placed, progressive increase in urine output
b. Patient treated with high-dose corticosteroids and dialysis. Creatinine slowly decreased to 1.2 mg/dl over next 3 weeks.

---

[a]SG = specific gravity

c. Offending medication(s) stopped; prednisone instituted; gradual return of renal function
d. Offending medication(s) stopped; Scr decreased to 1.8 mg/dl
e. Normal saline was administered at 200 cc/hr with urine output increasing to 50 cc/hr in 24 hr.
f. Hemodialysis instituted; renal function begins to return in about 4 weeks

Diagnosis:

a. Obstructive uropathy 2°, prostatic hypertrophy
b. Acute (allergic) interstitial nephritis
c. Diffuse proliferative GN due to systemic lupus erythematosus
d. ATN due to sepsis
e. Prerenal azotemia due to "third spacing"
f. Acute renal insufficiency 2° drug-induced vasomotor reaction in presence of bilateral renal artery stenosis.

chapter 10

Chronic Renal Failure

Pavel Vancura and Bruce S. Chang

Many chronic renal diseases progressively damage the kidneys and produce chronic renal failure (CRF). This usually has an asymptomatic stage marked by slowly worsening renal function and an end stage marked by uremic symptoms, debilitation and, in the absence of treatment, death. Up to 40–50% of patients presenting with **end stage renal disease (ESRD)** are not aware of any preexisting renal disease. Consequently, the news that they have ESRD is a "shock" and understandably gives rise to fear, anger, depression or denial. The impact of chronic renal failure is not only a personal one, but is a major drain on the human and financial resources of our nation's health care system. The present treatment for ESRD involves high technology dialysis and transplantation. These methods are imperfect, expensive and with about 100,000 patients on chronic dialysis in the United States cost the federal government each year about $2 billion.

Definitions

Renal failure means loss of GFR. It can be qualified as mild, moderate, or severe or better still, it can be quantified with the values of Scr or Ccr. The adjectives **chronic** or **acute** add the dimension of time.

Furthermore, chronic implies irreversibility. A variety of kidney diseases can lead to CRF (see Etiology). They may be stable or progressive and can leave the patient with a spectrum of GFR's ranging from the mildest impairment to life-threatening loss of function. As the kidneys fail and nephrons "drop out", we may see an increase in the size and GFR of the remaining nephrons, as well as compensatory adjustments of the body and kidneys to the decreased renal function. These adaptations are limited, however, and with progressive renal damage a clinical syndrome called **uremia** develops.

Etiology

The underlying etiology in almost half of patients with CRF is one of the forms of GN. The next most important cause is diabetic nephropathy, accounting for 20% of patients; several other diseases are responsible for the remaining cases (Table 10.1).

Pathogenesis

For several renal conditions listed above such as chronic GN, diabetic nephropathy or polycystic kidneys, it is easy to understand how the ongoing disease process produces pathologic changes leading to a decrease in renal mass and GFR. However, in certain disorders, even after the primary insult or noxious agent is eliminated, renal function continues to decline due to progressive sclerosis of glomeruli. It is proposed that following the initial loss of nephrons hyperperfusion and hyperfiltration take place in the remaining glomeruli in order to compensate for reduced GFR. This leads to increased permeation of albumin into the mesangial areas and to gradual glomerulosclerosis and renal failure in the absence of activity of the underlying renal disease (see chapter on **renal perfusion disorders**). It is possible that this process also exacerbates the ongoing damage in those diseases such as chronic GN with continued disease activity.

Clinical Features

The clinical manifestations of the uremic syndrome develop as the various renal functions fail. Recalling that the kidney performs excretory, regulatory and hormonal functions, we will examine the impact of renal failure on each.

Table 10.1.
Principal Causes of Chronic Renal Failure

I. Glomerular
   A. Any chronic GN (primary or multisystem disease, e.g., systemic lupus erythematosus)
   B. Diabetic nephropathy
   C. Amyloidosis
   D. Alport's disease
II. Vascular
   A. Hypertensive nephrosclerosis
   B. Bilateral renal artery stenosis
III. Obstructive uropathy
   A. Tumors
   B. Benign prostatic hypertrophy
   C. Neurogenic bladder
IV. Tubulointerstitial
   A. Polycystic kidney disease
   B. Myeloma kidney

Excretory Function

A number of substances come into the body as part of the diet. Some are excreted unchanged; others are converted to metabolic waste products. In either case one can think of the substances as representing a "load" which the kidneys must excrete in order to maintain balance, or homeostasis. As the kidneys lose GFR, due to a progressive loss of nephrons, the surviving nephrons adjust in several ways to maintain waste excretion.

Compensatory Hypertrophy and Hyperperfusion of Surviving Nephrons. The first adjustment is enlargement, increased perfusion and increased "single nephron" GFR of the remaining nephrons. The ability of the kidney to hypertrophy is greatest in the young and declines with age. This phenomenon is readily observed in some individuals born with only one kidney. They have half as many nephrons as someone with two kidneys, but they have a GFR indistinguishable from normal. It is also seen in the remaining tissue when one surgically removes part of a kidney or a whole kidney, and when a disease causes patchy injury to the kidneys.

Increased Plasma Concentration of Substance. A second compensatory change is to sustain excretion through increasing the concentration of the substance in the plasma. Chapter 1 **(review of normal renal physiology)** described how reductions of Ccr are followed by a rise in

Scr until creatinine excretion again matches production. Urea and a host of other nitrogenous substances are handled similarly by the kidney and declining GFR leads to increases in their serum concentrations. With severe renal failure certain substances normally excreted in the urine build up to what are felt to be toxic levels, thereby producing the symptoms of uremia (urine in the blood, see section on **specific symptoms** below). These affect the neuromuscular, gastrointestinal and other systems. The identification of these uremic toxins has been the subject of much unsuccessful investigation. Urea and creatinine are apparently not noxious enough to be the culprits. However, other compounds that accumulate in CRF, including organic degradation products, enzymes, hormones and peptides, are now under suspicion. Also the clearance of many renally excreted drugs is reduced in CRF, raising their serum concentrations occasionally to toxic levels.

Regulatory Function

Reduced Tubular Reabsorption of Sodium and Water. An important adaptive mechanism in CRF is **diminished tubular reabsorption** of a highly reabsorbed substance. Normally large amounts of Na^+ and water filter through the glomeruli, but greater than 98–99% is reabsorbed. When GFR declines, a decreased fraction of the filtered Na^+ and water must be reabsorbed, which is to say an **increasing fraction** must be excreted for the organism to remain in balance. This adaptation for Na^+ was depicted in Figure 2.1. In this way, most patients with CRF are able to maintain a urine output of Na^+ and water to balance their daily intake. This capacity is often maintained until GFR reaches very low levels, less than 5–10 ml/min. How the kidney manages this increased fractional excretion of Na^+ is not clear. There is some suggestion that a humoral substance, such as atrial natriuretic factor, is responsible.

Although capable of maintaining balance for Na^+ and water, the kidney becomes much less flexible. While usual intakes of Na^+ and water are handled well, there is a limited response to large loads or sudden restrictions. Large Na^+ loads may precipitate hypervolemia and restriction may result in volume depletion due to salt wasting. In CRF both urinary dilution and concentration are also impaired. This may be due to the fact that relatively fewer nephrons in the inner cortex have the job of establishing the corticomedullary concentration gradient compared with the more abundant nephrons in the outer cortex which produce the bulk of the dilute urine for excretion.

Reduced Tubular Reabsorption of Phosphate. Another example of adjustment through increasing the fractional excretion is the renal handling of phosphorus. Phosphorus exists in plasma mainly as inorganic phosphate ion, either as HPO_4^{2-} or as $H_2PO_4^-$. Normal renal excretion of phosphate is about 10–20% of the filtered amount. With progressive decreases in GFR and filtered phosphate, the fractional excretion rises to between 40–50% and can increase to 90–100% at GFR of less than 10 ml/min. Increased secretion of parathormone (PTH) acts on the renal tubule to reduce phosphate reabsorption. This mechanism is able to maintain a normal serum phosphorus level (2–4 mg/dl), often until GFR is about 30 ml/min; below that one begins to see elevation of serum phosphorus. Thus the patient with less than 30 ml/min GFR still excretes a daily phosphorus load of about 1 gm, but does so by decreasing tubular reabsorption **and** by increasing the filtered load per nephron (Fig. 10.1).

Trade-Off Hypothesis. It is appropriate here to mention a concept, that each of these adjustments occurs at some cost to the organism, i.e., a **trade-off** takes place. The renal handling of phosphate is a paradigm: as GFR decreases, there is a tendency for the serum phosphorus to rise. Because of a biochemical balance between phosphate and ionized Ca^{2+}, a rise in the former tends to lower the latter. Lower ionized Ca^{2+} concentration is sensed by the parathyroid gland as a signal to increase secretion of PTH (Fig. 10.2). This hormone then maintains the level of ionized Ca^{2+} through increased bone resorption, which releases Ca^{2+} into the circulation and also through increased renal reabsorption of filtered Ca^{2+}. Along with this PTH promotes the excretion of phosphate, and thereby maintains the serum concentration at normal levels. Thus, increased PTH secretion is able to maintain the balance of phosphate in CRF, but there is a trade-off. The trade-off for the increased excretion of phosphate is higher PTH secretion, greater bone resorption and secondary bone disease. Thus, adjustments to an increasingly abnormal internal environment may inevitably favor some systems at the expense of others. The ultimate example of this is the increased single nephron GFR that helps compensate for nephron loss and may itself produce glomerular sclerosis and further nephron loss.

Increased Secretion. Another way the kidney can increase excretion of a substance as the filtered amount decreases is to increase secretion. This is the mechanism that maintains K^+ homeostasis until very low GFRs are reached. Current concepts of the renal handling of K^+ hold

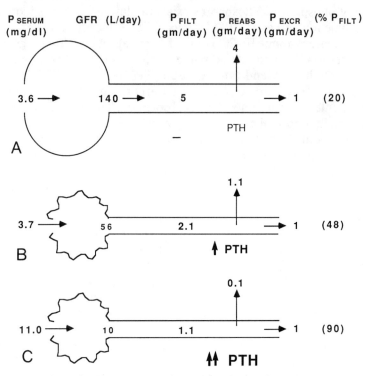

Figure 10.1.   Maintenance of phosphate excretion in the face of diminishing GFR. (A) Normal GFR. (B) 60% loss of GFR: phosphate excretion maintained by reduced tubular reabsorption. (C) 93% loss of GFR: phosphate excretion maintained by further reduction in tubular reabsorption and increased serum level. Role of PTH in reducing tubular reabsorption is shown.

that virtually all of the excreted K^+ is secreted in the distal nephron, normally 80–120 mEq/day. This is about 10% of the filtered amount. At very low GFR the excreted K^+ may even exceed the amount filtered, as long as urine volume is adequate. This remarkable achievement is evidence that urinary K^+ is secreted. Increased aldosterone levels may be responsible for the increased tubular K^+ secretion, but the data are unclear on this point. Increased secretion of creatinine has also been observed, but this has little clinical relevance. One might

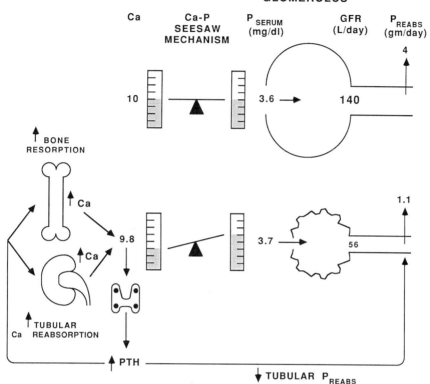

Figure 10.2. Role of hypocalcemia and increased PTH secretion in regulation of phosphate balance in CRF. Upper mechanism represents normal renal function. Lower nephron represents CRF. High phosphate concentration lowers Ca^{2+} concentration which stimulates parathyroid glands to secrete PTH. The higher PTH levels act on the renal tubules to lower serum phosphate concentration and on the renal tubules and bone to increase serum Ca^{2+} concentration.

expect that such augmented secretory capacity may hold for other organic compounds, including certain drugs.

For some substances balance is maintained by increasing **excretion via nonrenal routes.** Intestinal secretion of uric acid and K^+ are examples.

The case of H^+ deserves comment because balance is not maintained and yet severe acidosis does not usually occur. The kidney may be able to secrete more H^+ per nephron, but there are insufficient buffers in the tubular fluid in advanced renal failure to take advantage of this. Specifically, there is insufficient generation of ammonia due to the loss of renal parenchymal cells. Severe acidosis is probably averted by the slow exchange of H^+ for Ca^{2+} in bone.

Hormonal Function

Erythropoietin. One might expect in CRF with loss of nephron mass and functioning renal parenchymal cells that production of erythropoietin may be decreased. Recent evidence has suggested that the erythropoietin secretion is not low, but high, although not as high as one might expect for the level of anemia. This relative insufficiency of erythropoietin leads to less than optimal bone marrow production of red cells, and along with decreased survival of red cells (see below) causes the anemia of CRF.

1,25-Dihydroxycholecalciferol. Active vitamin D can legitimately be considered a renal hormone. The hydroxylation at the 1 position of 1,25-dihydroxycholecalciferol takes place in the kidney and it is through the regulation of this hydroxylation step that the regulation of gastrointestinal absorption of Ca^{2+} is accomplished. In severe CRF 1,25-dihydroxycholecalciferol levels are depressed. Along with high serum phosphate they lead to hypocalcemia and the secondary hyperparathyroidism mentioned above.

Renin. Renin secretion takes place in the damaged kidney much as in the normal kidney; however, its regulation may not be the same. In some kidney diseases renin secretion appears to be inappropriately high or low. High renin states may contribute to hypertension through the increased production of angiotensin II. In other patients, excess extracellular volume causes hypertension, which in turn lowers renin secretion, and ultimately aldosterone levels. As a result, tubular secretion of K^+ and H^+ is impaired, leading to hyperkalemia and acidosis. The mechanisms involved in this disorder called **hyporeninemic hypoaldosteronism** are still being investigated.

Stages of Chronic Renal Failure

As the biochemical environment deteriorates with decreasing GFR, changes inevitably occur in a variety of organ systems. The typical patient with progressive CRF may be considered to pass through four clinical stages (Fig. 10.3).

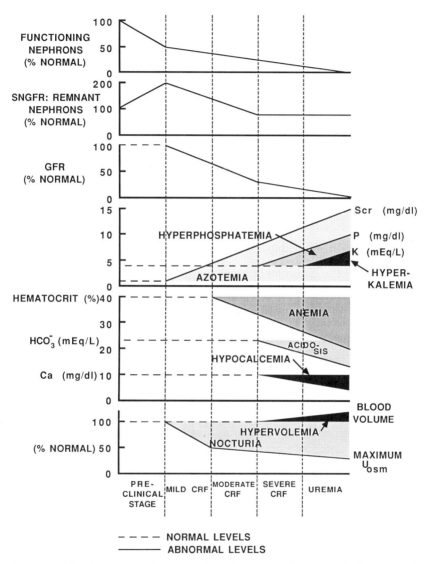

Figure 10.3. Depiction of the preclinical stage and four clinical stages of chronic renal failure. In the preclinical stage increasing single nephron GFR offsets the loss of nephrons and maintains renal function. SNGFR = single nephron GFR. (Modified from Fine LG: Hosp Pract 22:59, 1987.)

The first stage is mild CRF (Scr normal–2.5 mg/dl; GFR 50–79 ml/min). The excretory and regulatory functions of the kidney are well preserved or minimally affected. Often at least half of normal function may be lost before the BUN or Scr rises above normal.

The second stage is moderate CRF and is manifested by mild azotemia (Scr 2.6–6.0 mg/dl; GFR 20–49 ml/min), inability to concentrate urine, nocturia and mild anemia. In this precarious state challenges such as catabolic illnesses or acute volume deficit, which would produce a barely recognizable alteration in Scr in a normal subject, may lead to severe azotemia and decompensation of previously adequate regulatory mechanisms.

The third stage is severe CRF (Scr 6.1–10 mg/dl; GFR 10–19 ml/min). Advanced anemia, hypocalcemia, hyperphosphatemia, metabolic acidosis, isosthenuria and nocturia are present. Sodium homeostasis is impaired and mild-to-moderate edema is common.

The fourth and final stage is **uremia** (Scr > 10 mg/dl; GFR < 10 ml/min). At this point all of the consequences of renal failure come to bear on the patient. The most common symptoms involve the gastrointestinal tract, the cardiovascular system, neuromuscular system and hematopoietic system. In addition, bone changes and endocrine abnormalities can develop.

Specific Symptoms

The major symptoms of uremia are listed on Table 10.2.

Gastrointestinal Symptoms. These are anorexia, nausea, vomiting and a foul taste in the mouth. Gastrointestinal symptoms are related to the degree of azotemia. It was stated in the first chapter that the BUN is influenced by protein intake as well as by GFR. Clinically, it has been observed that reducing the BUN and presumably other breakdown products by restricting protein intake can relieve many of the GI symptoms despite an unchanged GFR.

Cardiovascular Symptoms. Heart failure due to hypervolemia is common. The patient is breathless and edematous. Hypertension and its consequences can be seen, including cerebrovascular accidents and coronary heart disease. Pericarditis can cause chest pain and an effusion, which may be large enough to cause cardiac tamponade.

Neuromuscular Symptoms. The common symptoms include lethargy, fatigue, a loss of ability to concentrate on complex tasks and a reversal of the usual sleep pattern, i.e. insomnia at night and sleeping during the day. The patients often report "restless legs," a vague feeling

Table 10.2.
Principal Uremic Symptoms

I.   Gastrointestinal
   A. Anorexia, nausea, vomiting
   B. Dysguesia (abnormal taste)
II. Cardiac
   A. Volume overload
   B. Pericarditis, tamponade
III. Neuromuscular
   A. Lethargy, fatigue
   B. Inability to concentrate
   C. Reversal of sleep
   D. Restless legs
   E. Convulsions
   F. Stupor, coma
   G. Peripheral neuropathy
IV. Hematologic
   A. Anemia
   B. Bleeding due to a platelet defect
V.   Bone
   A. Pain
   B. Pathological fractures
   C. Impaired growth
VI. Endocrine
   A. Amenorrhea
   B. Reduced libido
   C. Reduced fertility
   D. Low sex hormone levels
VII. Dermatologic-itching

---

of discomfort in the legs when at rest that compels frequent changes in position to seek relief. A peripheral neuropathy may be seen, which results in atrophy and weakness of distal muscle groups, and loss of distal sensation. Severe uremia may cause hyperirritability in the neuromuscular systems beginning as hyperactive reflexes and ending as convulsions. In the most advanced cases, the patient may develop stupor or coma. The hyperactivity appears to be due to instability of neuromuscular membranes, while neuropathy is associated with axonal degeneration and secondary demyelination.

Hematologic Symptoms. Anemia and a tendency to bleed are the main problems observed. The bleeding tendency is due primarily to a defect in platelet function, while platelet number is normal. Although there may be several causes of the anemia, it is mainly due to mild hemolysis coupled with an impaired bone marrow response. The cause of hemolysis is not well understood, but is probably multifactorial. Red cell survival is shortened. Relative deficiency of erythropoietin impairs marrow response to anemia and was commented upon above. Also blood loss, often from the gastrointestinal tract, aggravates the anemia. The degree of anemia is not closely correlated to the degree of chronic renal failure. Hematocrits may range from near normal to 20%, at which point anemia contributes to the reduced stamina. The anemia is usually normochromic, but many bizarre red cells can be seen in the blood.

Bone Symptoms. Less noticeable to the patient, but in time obvious to the physician, is the problem of bone disease in CRF. There are two components usually: first, the excessive breakdown or resorption of bone because of excessive secretion of PTH and, secondly, poor mineralization of newly formed bone due to lack of Ca^{2+}, which is the result of inadequate production of active vitamin D (Fig. 10.4). The combination is referred to as **renal osteodystrophy.** Bone pain and pathological fractures may be seen. In children, growth is retarded. Frequently the bones appear minimally changed or even normal on roentgenography, but examination of a biopsied specimen will show evidence of bone disease in virtually all patients with CRF.

Endocrine Symptoms. Sexual function is profoundly affected in adults of both sexes with ESRD. In female patients, menstrual periods often cease and even moderate CRF leads to lowered fertility and increased rate of spontaneous abortion. The risk of toxemia is greatly increased. Males are subfertile and libido is reduced in both sexes. Testosterone, estrogen and progesterone levels may be low.

Dermatologic Symptoms. One of the most vexing uremic symptoms is itching. It may become intolerable. The reasons for this severe itching are not understood, but it may be related to urea, uric acid and Ca^{2+} deposits in the skin, and to salt and water loss making skin dry.

Treatment

A conservative therapeutic approach may be adequate for a spectrum of patients from those with only moderate CRF to those with a GFR as low as 10 ml/min. On the other hand, when CRF progresses to ESRD, so little renal function remains that aggressive therapy such as peritoneal dialysis, hemodialysis or renal transplantation is necessary.

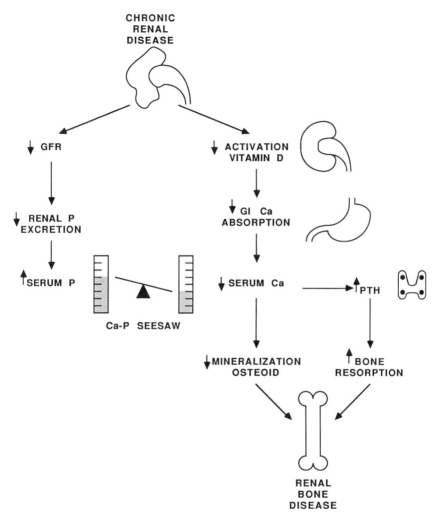

Figure 10.4. Schematic representation of the pathogenesis of renal osteodystrophy.

Conservative Approach

The management of patients with CRF should ideally counteract the adverse effects of diminishing renal function and should prevent further loss of renal mass. The conservative approach decreases the burden imposed on the kidney by reducing the load on the system. One can adjust the intakes of Na^+, K^+, water, phosphorus and protein to the amount of residual GFR. Fortunately, Na^+, water and K^+ balance are remarkably well preserved until severe renal failure, so that initially their dietary intake need not be restricted. It is more important to restrict protein and phosphate intake and to bind phosphorus in the gastrointestinal tract by administering aluminum or Ca^{2+} salts. The low protein diet relieves some of the manifestations of uremia and reducing phosphate absorption prevents or mitigates the bone disease of CRF.

Protein restriction may have to be as low as 20 gm/day or about 25% of the normal Western diet. Malnutrition is avoided because the body is capable of synthesizing nonessential amino acids from carbohydrates by amination. Urea is metabolized by bowel bacteria, releasing ammonia, which is used to convert ketoacids to amino acids. As long as adequate essential amino acids are provided as part of the 20-gm protein diet, the patient can be maintained in nitrogen balance. The chief obstacle to this approach is unpalatability of the diet; consequently, in the United States low protein diets are mainly used to control uremic symptoms for short periods until dialysis may be conveniently started.

Administration of Ca^{2+} salts and analogs of vitamin D that do not require renal activation improves low intestinal absorption of Ca^{2+} and reverses poor bone mineralization.

With certain exceptions like correcting chronic obstruction or controlling hypertension in diabetics, we cannot unequivocally slow or prevent progression of CRF. Research is currently evaluating the efficacy of low protein diets, ACE inhibitors and other modalities in slowing progression of CRF.

Dialytic Approach (Optional Reading)

There comes a time when uremic symptoms occur despite limitation of intake and some way must be found to maintain water and electrolyte homeostasis and to remove the metabolic wastes from the body. Dialysis has become the most widely used therapy for patients with ESRD. Chronic dialysis may sustain life long term (?decades) even in anephric patients. The same dialysis procedure, referred to in this case as acute dialysis, is used in patients with acute renal failure for one to several weeks until recovery of renal function takes place.

Principles of Dialysis. Dialysis is defined as the transfer of solutes across a semipermeable membrane (one which permits the passage of molecules smaller than a few thousand daltons in size, such as urea or Na^+, but no large molecules, such as proteins, or formed elements such as red cells, white cells or bacteria). The principle is old, but the application has only been exploited since the 1960s, when reliable methods of access to the circulation, a suitable anticoagulant, heparin, and biocompatible plastics and polymers were introduced. The membrane can be **synthetic,** as in the case of the "artificial kidney" used in hemodialysis, or **natural** as in the case of peritoneal membrane used in peritoneal dialysis.

During dialysis any substance in solution tends to move from regions where it is in high concentration to regions where it is in low concentration. This is a consequence of random diffusion of the molecules. In both peritoneal dialysis and hemodialysis the blood is brought into contact with a solution, dialysate, from which it is separated by a membrane. The small molecules will travel across the membrane down the concentration gradient, into or out of the blood, depending upon the concentration difference between blood and dialysate. By adjusting the composition of the dialysate any small molecular weight substance can be made to enter or leave the patient during dialysis, or to remain in equilibrium. This is true of any naturally occurring molecule, and also of drugs and poisons. During dialysis, metabolic wastes, most of which are under 1000 daltons in size, diffuse out of the blood into the dialysate where their concentration is zero. Potassium, phosphate and sulfate derived from the diet are also dialyzed out, while HCO_3^- is **dialyzed in** in order to correct acidosis. In this way, the excretory and regulatory functions of the kidney may be replaced, although rather clumsily.

There remains one problem, water. Generally, patients with oliguria gain 0.5–1 kg/day in water. One can think of water as being dissolved in its solutes. The concentration of water is greatest where the solution is dilute and the concentration of water is low in strong solutions, where the osmolarity is high. Water tends to flow in the direction of the concentration gradient. In order to remove water from the patient, we may make the dialysate more concentrated than the patient's blood. High concentration is especially exploited in peritoneal dialysis, where we raise the osmotic pressure of the dialysate with glucose to "suck" water out of the patient. We can also use hydrostatic pressure to remove water. Water will move across a membrane according to hydrostatic pressure differences. In hemodialysis, we "pull" water out of the patient by raising the hydrostatic pressure of the blood or applying negative pressure or suction to the dialysate. This process is called ultrafiltration.

Peritoneal Dialysis. Peritoneal dialysis, because of its relative simplicity, is frequently used in clinical practice for both acute and chronic renal failure. The peritoneal lining with its rich supply of blood is well suited as a dialysis membrane. After introduction of a sterile dialysis catheter into the peritoneal cavity, dialysate (most commonly 2 L) prewarmed to the body temperature is run in, left for about 30 minutes in the peritoneal cavity for dialysis to occur and then drained (Fig. 10.5). After this another 2 L of dialysis fluid is run in and the procedure is repeated hourly for 36–48 hours. A modification of peritoneal dialysis called chronic ambulatory peritoneal dialysis or CAPD is widely used for patients with ESRD.

Hemodialysis. In hemodialysis, the process of dialysis takes place through a membrane in a dialyzer (artificial kidney). Dialyzers may differ as to manufacturer, size and material and configuration of the membrane. For example, parallel sheets of cellulose may be used or "hollow fibers" of Cupraphane. A great variety of dialyzers are available. What is common for all of them is the fact that a small volume of blood is presented over a maximum surface area of a membrane, washed on the other side with the dialyzing fluid. Blood taken from the patient is pumped through dialysis blood lines (plastic tubing) into the dialyzer and then back into the patient. To prevent blood clotting in the system, the patient receives heparin during the treatment. Several monitoring devices in the system, such as a blood leak detector, help assure the safety of the procedure. The dialysate delivery system prepares the dialysate by mixing water with a concentrated solution of solutes, heats the dialysate to body

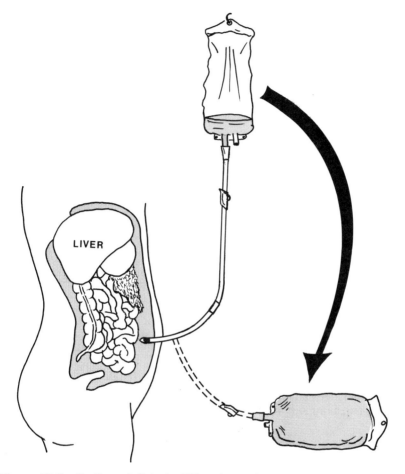

Figure 10.5. Peritoneal dialysis. Filling the peritoneal space with dialysate and subsequent draining by raising and lowering dialysate bag.

temperature and pumps it through the dialyzer at an adjustable flow rate and pressure (Fig. 10.6).

In hemodialysis, some means of access to the patient's circulation is needed to facilitate the removal and return of blood. For chronic dialysis, a surgeon creates a subcutaneous arteriovenous (A-V) fistula in the upper extremity by anastamosing an artery and a vein or by inserting a length of arti-

DIALYSATE DELIVERY SYSTEM

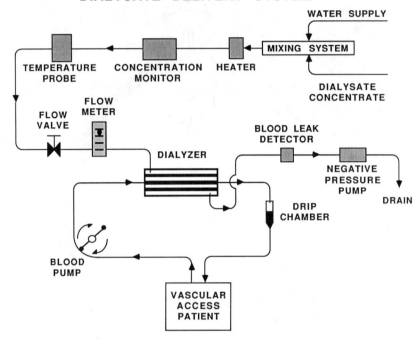

EXTRACORPOREAL BLOOD CIRCUIT

Figure 10.6. Schematic diagram of hemodialysis. Both the dialysis delivery system and extracorporeal blood circuit are shown.

ficial vessel (a vascular graft) between an artery and a vein. The A-V fistula must "mature" for about 2 weeks, after which the patient has a large subcutaneous high flow blood vessel into which needles may be easily inserted. For acute dialysis, a catheter in the subclavian or femoral vein provides quick access to the circulation.

A patient normally undergoes hemodialysis for 3–4 hours at a time 3 times a week.

Dialysis should not be seen as returning the patient to normal renal function. **It does not.** In general, the patient on dialysis attains a level of function comparable to a GFR of 15–20 ml/min. Although the gastrointestinal and neurologic symptoms are dramatically reduced, some of the problems of uremia remain, such as anemia and endocrine abnormalities. Children do not grow well and they fail to mature normally, both physically and psychologically. Women continue with abnormal menses and remain infertile. Men are often impotent. Although many patients return to full employment, others, because of easy fatigability or other illness, achieve only partial rehabilitation. Survival of more than 10 years on chronic dialysis is not unusual, but life expectancy does not return to normal.

Renal Transplantation (Optional Reading)

When successful, this approach brings a patient closest to normal. The most successful recipients of kidney transplants take only a few pills a day, see their doctor occasionally, and lead as normal a life as their general health will allow. The surgical procedure of transplanting the kidney from one person to another is routinely performed without difficulty. The source of the graft may be from a close blood relative or from an unrelated cadaver. Kidneys from the latter group are maintained in a sterile, chilled state up to 72 hours, while the recipient is selected and prepared for transplantation.

Immunologic Rejection. A major obstacle to universal application of this therapy is the rejection of the graft by the recipient's immune system. It has become apparent that at least two factors are important in achieving graft tolerance: the immunologic response of the recipient and antigenic similarity between donor and recipient. Antigenic compatibility is sought as follows: The donor and recipient must be blood group ABO compatible. The major histocompatibility antigens, so-called HLA (human leukocyte antigen) antigens, are identified from the leukocytes of both donor and recipient. An attempt is made to select a donor with many, if not all, HLA antigens identical to that of the recipient. A good match between recipient and donor favors a good outcome. The fact that poorly matched transplants still may survive suggests that the degree of recipient response to grafting may be important, and the fact that apparently perfectly matched transplants sometimes fail suggests that there is more to our antigenic makeup than these HLA antigens alone.

Immunosuppressive Therapy. The most important complication of the renal transplant is the **rejection** of the graft, in which cells, antibodies and a host of secondary mechanisms, including complement and platelets, destroy the allograft. In the management of rejection of the graft, we attempt to prevent or blunt the rejection reaction. Various agents are used to minimize the reaction of the recipient to the foreign kidney. These inhibit the immunologic defense mechanisms and are called **immunosuppressive drugs.** They include synthetic **corticosteroid** hormones (usually prednisone), **azathioprine,** which was originally synthesized as an anticancer agent, and **cyclosporin A,** a fungal metabolite. **Antilymphocyte globulin** containing antibodies to lymphocyte antigens may produce effective immunologic suppression on a temporary basis and is used to treat acute rejection. These drugs are currently used to achieve tolerance to the graft, but unfortunately they also reduce the defenses of the patient against a hostile microbial environment. Although modern immunosuppressive therapy has unquestionably improved the survival of the transplanted kidney and patient, death from bacterial, fungal or viral infections remains a major risk.

Long-Term Results. Living related donor transplants, i.e., between parents and children or between siblings and especially between identical twins, have a higher chance of success than cadaver donor transplants. At 2 years related donor grafts have a 90% chance of functioning, while cadaveric grafts have about a 80% chance and the gap widens with the time. Nevertheless, cadaveric grafts may be the only possible source for many patients and constitute 60% of the total renal transplantations. Long-term successes of both types of transplant, greater than 10 years, are not rare, but chronic rejection takes a significant toll as does occasional return of the original disease to the transplanted kidney. In addition to the graft rejection, patients with renal transplantation face the problem of complications of immunosuppressant therapy. Systemic infection may occur in any patient maintained on immunosuppressives and the infective agents can be bacterial (mostly gram negative bacteria), viruses (cytomegalovirus, varicella and hepatitis), fungi (aspergillus and nocardia), yeast (candida and cryptococcus), and protozoa (pneumocystis carinii). Other complications seen are Cushing's syndrome, secondary to corticosteroid therapy, and also malignant tumors, especially lymphomas, which have an increased incidence. Despite these dangers, successes of transplantation can be impressive. Patients achieve a feeling of well-being that is lacking on dialysis. Children grow and mature, men father children and women conceive and deliver healthy babies.

Suggested Readings

Anagnostou A. The hematologic disorders of chronic renal failure. Semin Nephrol 1985;5:79–197.

Eknoyan G. Chronic renal failure. Semin Nephrol 1981;1:87–198.

Fine LG. The uremic syndrome: Adaptive mechanisms and therapy. Hosp Pract 1987;22:59–69.

Giordano C. IV Capri Conference on uremia. Kidney Int 1985;28(S17):S1–S188.

Hull AR. Dialysis and transplantation: The view from the 80s. Semin Nephrol 1982;2:75–186.

Klahr S, Schreiner G, Ichikawa I. The progression of renal disease. NEJM 1988;318:1657–1666.

Malangone JM, Abuelo JG, Pezzullo JC, Lund K, McGloin CA. Clinical and laboratory features of patients at the start of chronic dialysis. Clin Nephrol, in press, 1989.

Massry SO, Kopple JD. Symposium on uremic toxins. Semin Nephrol 1983;3:261–395.

Nolph KD, Lindblad AS, Novak JW. Continuous ambulatory peritoneal dialysis. NEJM 1988;318:1595–1600.

Stone WJ, Rabin PL. End-stage renal disease. An integrated approach. New York, Academic Press Inc., 1983.

CHRONIC RENAL FAILURE PROBLEMS

1. A 35-year-old man is referred to your office because of anorexia, nausea, itching and weakness lasting for 2 months. Physical examination shows weight loss of 7 kg; skin is pale and there is 1+ pitting edema around the ankles. Otherwise the examination is unremarkable. Blood tests reveal BUN 138 and Scr 12.9 mg/dl. In this clinical setting the blood or serum concentrations of each of the following substances might be abnormal. Indicate for each substance whether you would expect a rise or fall from normal or if either could be seen.
   A. Na^+
   B. K^+
   C. HCO_3^-
   D. Hemoglobin
   E. Aldosterone
   F. Ca^{2+}
   G. Phosphate
   H. PTH

   I. Erythropoietin

   J. Renin

2. Your patient's serum phosphate is 7.5 mg/dl and his serum Ca^{2+} is 7.9 mg/dl. X-ray films of his feet and hands show a mild degree of bone disease of CRF.

   A. This condition is caused by (choose all that are applicable):

      a. Increase secretion of PTH

      b. Anemia

      c. Hyponatremia

      d. Inadequate production of active vitamin D

      e. High BUN

   B. You might consider treating the patient's renal bone disease with all of the following **EXCEPT**:

      a. Binding of phosphorus in the gut with aluminum salt

      b. Administration of active analog of vitamin D and Ca^{2+} salts

      c. Ask an orthopedic surgeon to perform bone surgery

      d. Avoid foods with high phosphate content

3. A 46-year-old woman on chronic dialysis for the last 2 years complains of periodic fatigue and mild shortness of breath. Her laboratory studies show BUN 98 mg/dl, Scr 9.3 mg/dl, Na^+ 128 mEq/L, K^+ 5.3 mEq/L, HCO_3^- 19 mEq/L, hemoglobin 6.7 g/dl and hematocrit 20%. EKG shows a premature ventricular contraction. Her symptoms are likely due to (choose one best answer):

   a. Premature ventricular contractions

   b. Normocytic normochromic anemia

   c. HCO_3^- 19 mEq/L secondary to metabolic acidosis

   d. Hyponatremia

   e. Hyperkalemia

4. For each substance in column A select the principal mechanism used by the body in CRF to maintain homeostasis or excretion.

Column A	Column B
1. Creatinine	a. Increased intestinal secretion
2. Water	b. Increased tubular secretion
3. Phosphorus	c. Reduced tubular reabsorption
4. Ca^{2+}	d. Increased erythropoietin
5. Uric acid	e. Release from the bone
6. K^+	f. Uptake by the bone
7. Hemoglobin	g. Increased plasma level
8. H^+	h. Decreased hemolysis

chapter 11

Urinalysis

J. Gary Abuelo

The urinalysis is a combination of **more or less unrelated urine tests,** that are performed because they **allow screening for common problems or disease,** e.g.

Appearance—hematuria, infection (pyuria)

Protein—all renal disease

Glucose—diabetes mellitus

Ketones—diabetes mellitus, starvation

Sediment—all renal disease (the most important element in this regard is red cells) or because they are **quick and inexpensive to perform:**

specific gravity

pH

A routine urinalysis is ordered for many kinds of patients:

1. Patients with suspected kidney disease
2. Patients with known kidney disease coming for a follow-up visit
3. Patients hospitalized for whatever reason
4. Patients seen in the doctor's office for any illness
5. Apparently well people getting routine checkups for camp, school teams, life insurance, new employment or school. (The need for urinalyses in asymptomatic children and adults under the ages of 30–40 is questionable, although it is a commonly performed test in this setting.)

Appearance

Fresh normal urine is usually clear. The color may vary from "straw" in a dilute urine to yellow in the average urine to slightly amber in a concentrated urine. As cooling to room temperature or to refrigerator temperature occurs, urates (in acid urine) or phosphates (in alkaline urine) may precipitate out, leading to a visible sediment or cloudy appearance.

Several abnormalities in appearance may be noted in various situations:

Red or Red-Brown Urine. This usually indicates the presence of blood and may be confirmed on examination of the urine sediment. If red cells are not seen, then the color is due to pigments, such as those found in patients eating beets (genetically susceptible individuals), taking certain drugs or having hemoglobin or myoglobin in the urine following hemolysis or muscle destruction.

Yellow-Brown Urine. This is usually due to excessive bilirubin in the urine and is a sign of liver disease.

Other Colors. Colors such as blue, green, purple, etc. may be due to breakdown products of drugs or abnormal metabolites of the body.

Cloudy Urine. If not due to precipitation of crystals on cooling, a cloudy appearance may be due to bacteria and white cells in urinary tract infections, red cells (smokey urine) or contamination of the urine with semen or fecal material.

Odor

Fresh normal urine has a faint odor. Infected urines may emit a fetid ammoniacal odor that is even noted by the patient. Certain metabolic disorders, such as maple syrup disease, lead to distinctive odors.

pH

The pH of the normal urine may vary from 4.5 to 8.0 depending on the acidity and alkalinity of the diet. Meat protein breaks down to acidic end products, while certain fruits and vegetables break down to alkaline end products. On the usual American diet, the urine pH is about 6. Urine pH is measured by indicator paper on the routine urinalysis. A pH meter may be used when performing special tests for renal tubular acidosis.

The urine pH is of interest to the clinician in just a few situations:

1. When certain bacteria infect the urine they elaborate urease, which releases NH_3 from the urea in the urine. A very high pH is produced (7.5–9.0) and kidney stones may be formed. Thus, the urine pH may be useful in determining the etiology of kidney stones.

2. Patients with metabolic or respiratory acidosis should excrete an acid urine (pH<5.5) in an effort to correct themselves. The absence of an acid urine in such a patient indicates the failure of urine acidification and suggests that the acidosis is due to renal tubular acidosis.

3. Patients with respiratory or metabolic alkalosis should produce an alkaline urine. The finding of an acid urine in such circumstances (paradoxical aciduria) usually indicates high rates of tubular $NaHCO_3$ reabsorption and H^+ secretion due to high levels of mineralocorticoids. Diagnoses of volume depletion with high renin and secondary high aldosterone levels (usually due to vomiting or diuretics) or primary mineralocorticoid excess states should be suspected (see chapter on **acid-base disorders**).

4. Patients with certain drug intoxications such as aspirin overdose are usually treated by alkalinizing their urine, which greatly increases urinary elimination of the drug. $NaHCO_3$ or acetazolamide may be administered using urine pH as a guideline for therapy.

Specific Gravity

Specific gravity is the weight of a sample of fluid in grams divided by its volume in ml. Pure water has a specific gravity of 1.000. The more concentrated the urine is (i.e. the higher the osmolality) the higher is the amount of dissolved substances as measured by specific gravity. This relationship is close enough that specific gravity provides an index of urine concentration. Normally, the urine concentration may range from very dilute (50 mOsm/L, specific gravity ~1.001) to isotonic (300 mOsm/L, specific gravity ~1.009 to 1.010) to very concentrated (1200 mOsm/L, specific gravity ~1.034). Since about 600 mOsm of urea, salts and other metabolic products are excreted in a day, these levels correspond to 24-hour urine outputs of 12 L, 2 L and 0.5 L, respectively. Specific gravity determination is a part of the routine urinalysis and is useful clinically under certain circumstances:

1. The routine urinalysis includes a measurement of protein concentration and a microscopic examination of the urine sediment. If the urine is excessively dilute, the protein may be too dilute to be detected

and cells and other elements in the sediment may be too sparse to be seen. Therefore, a "reasonably" concentrated urine specimen, (specific gravity > 1.015) should be used for the urinalysis. The first morning specimen is generally preferred for routine urinalysis, because it tends to be concentrated. The routine inclusion of specific gravity gives the physician an idea of the dilution factor that he is dealing with.

2. In diagnosing polyuria, specific gravity will be low (<1.005) in loss of concentrating ability (diabetes insipidus) and psychogenic polydipsia and high (>1.020) in diabetes mellitus, in which the patient may be dehydrated but is undergoing an osmotic diuresis.

3. Patients with hypotension may have azotemia and a reduced GFR due to poor renal perfusion (prerenal azotemia) or they may have sustained ischemic damage to the tubules (acute tubular necrosis). The specific gravity may help distinguish between these two possibilities, being high (>1.020) in the first case and isotonic (∼1.010) in the second case.

Protein

Urine protein concentration is determined semiquantitatively as part of the urinalysis. Normal protein excretion is <150 mg/day, about half being filtered albumin and the other half being Tamm-Horsfall protein that is produced and secreted by the tubular cells. Assuming a normal urine volume of 1 L/day, the average protein concentration of the urine should be no more than 15 mg/dl. Proteinuria is detected with reagent strips that change color or with acids such as sulfosalicylic acid that form a visible protein precipitate on exposure to urine protein concentrations greater than 10–20 mg/dl. The color change or amount of turbidity can be graded from trace to 4+ with 3+ and 4+ corresponding usually to nephrotic range proteinuria (about 300–1000 mg/dl). If a positive protein test is obtained, a protein/creatinine ratio on a single urine specimen or a 24-hour urine for protein should be done to quantitate the proteinuria. Any renal disease can cause some proteinuria as can strenuous exercise, fever and congestive heart failure. Nephrotic range proteinuria suggests a glomerular lesion.

Glucose and Ketone

These tests are usually done with reagent strips as part of the routine urinalysis. They are mainly screening tests for diabetes mellitus. No glucose or ketones are detected in normal urine, while both are present in diabetic ketoacidosis. Glucose may also be seen with defective proximal tubular reabsorption of glucose (Fanconi's syndrome; see chapter on **acid-base disorders**); and ketones are excreted in starvation.

Blood

A reagent strip sensitive to peroxidase activity changes color when exposed to red cells, hemoglobin or myoglobin. Intravascular hemolysis causes hematuria, while muscle damage caused, for example, by a crush injury or strenuous exercise, gives rise to myoglobinuria. The detection of blood with a reagent strip should be verified by the observation of red cells on microscopy of the urine sediment.

Microscopic Examination of the Urinary Sediment

Ten or 15 ml of fresh urine are centrifuged; the supernatant is decanted, and the sediment is resuspended in the small amount of residual urine. A drop of this suspension is placed on a slide under a coverslip and examined with a microscope (Fig. 11.1). Casts are searched for under low power (10X objective) and are reported as rare, few or many. Cells are counted in 10 fields using the 40X objective and are reported as cells per high-power field (e.g. 3–5 red blood cells per high-power field or RBC/HPF).

Red Cells

Most individuals normally excrete in the urine up to 1 million red cells/day, which corresponds to about 1 RBC per 2 high-power fields (reported as "rare" or "occasional"). Individuals with between 1 and 4 RBC/HPF make up about 5% of the apparently healthy population. Clinically significant hematuria is 5 RBC/HPF or more. The entry point of red cells into normal urine is not known. In patients with hematuria, blood may enter the urine anywhere along the urinary tract from the glomerulus (glomerulonephritis) to the tip of the penis (bleeding circumcision). With menstruation, blood may contaminate the urine after it leaves the body. The causes of hematuria are multiple with infections, stones, tumors and glomerulonephritis being the most common etiologies. Transient hematuria may also be seen after strenuous exercise. Red cells in the urine may appear as spherical (dilute urine), crenated (concentrated urine) or as typical biconcave discs.

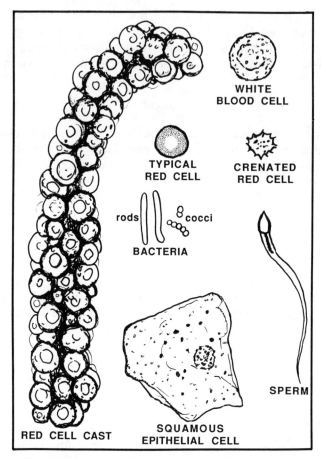

Figure 11.1. Examples of cells and other formed elements that can be found in the urine sediment.

White Cells

Up to 2 million white cells (WBC) are excreted in the urine per day. More than 4 WBC/HPF is considered abnormal. Inflammatory processes in the kidney and anywhere along the urinary tract may lead to increased urinary white cells (pyuria). The most common cause of large amounts of white cells in the urine is infection. White cells in the urine appear as granular spheres about 50% larger than red cells. The nuclei may or may not be visible.

Renal Tubular Cells

Renal tubular cells are 1–3 times the size of leukocytes and have large round nuclei. They often cannot be distinguished from white cells without special staining. Occasional renal tubular cells may be seen in normal urine. Increased numbers of these cells reflect active degeneration of the tubules and may be seen in acute renal disease such as acute tubular necrosis, pyelonephritis and glomerulonephritis.

Squamous Epithelial Cells

These cells are large and flat and have small nuclei. They slough off the bladder wall or often are contaminants from the vagina. Their appearance in the urine has no clinical significance.

Casts

Casts are masses of protein formed when the urinary protein gels and is molded by the tubular walls into a cylindrical shape. The bulk of the protein is Tamm-Horsfall protein, which is agglutinated by the presence of increased amounts of albumin. **Hyaline casts** consist of protein alone. **Granular casts** are thought to be formed by "granules" of serum proteins trapped in a matrix of Tamm-Horsfall proteins. Both hyaline and granular casts are occasionally seen in normals but occur in increased numbers in renal diseases characterized by proteinuria. Acute tubular necrosis often leads to the appearance of red-brown granular casts. **Red cell casts** usually imply the presence of glomerulonephritis although rarely they may be seen in nonglomerular renal diseases. **White cell casts** reflect acute inflammatory disease of the kidney and are not specific for any one condition. With the progression of renal disease to a chronic stage one may see wide casts called **broad casts** and homogeneous casts with sharp outlines, called **waxy casts.**

Bacteria

Bacteria are not observed in normal urine. When more than 1 bacterium/HPF is observed in a fresh urine it usually indicates a urinary tract infection. Cocci are difficult to identify with certainty on the routine microscopic examination. A Gram's stain or culture will confirm their presence.

Crystals

Crystals are commonly seen in the urine sediment, especially if the urine has cooled down. A variety of crystals may be identified from their typical shape; however, they are rarely of clinical significance.

Table 11.1.
Urinalysis Reports for Problems

Case	1	2	3	4	5	6	7
Color	Tea	Yellow	Red brown	Yellow	Straw	Yellow	Amber
Appearance	Smoky	Clear	Bloody	Clear	Clear	Cloudy	Clear
Specific gravity	1.020	1.015	1.020	1.010	1.028	1.030	1.031
pH	6	7	6	5	5	7.5	5
Protein	3+	—	2+	Trace	—	1+	1+
Glucose	—	1+	—	—	4+	—	—
Ketones	—	—	—	—	1+	—	1+
Blood	4+	—	4+	—	—	—	+
Sediment							
RBC/HPF	>100	—	—	—	—	—	5–10
WBC/HPF	1–2	—	—	—	—	—	0–1
Hyaline casts	Occ.	—	—	—	—	Occ.	Occ.
Granular casts	Occ.	—	Red brown	Many brown	—	—	Rare
Other casts	Occ. RBC	—	—	—	—	—	—
Epithelial cells	—	—	—	—	—	Few squamous	—
Bacteria	—	—	—	—	—	—	—
Crystals	—	—	—	—	—	Amorphous urates	Calcium oxalate
Fat	—	—	—	—	—	—	—
Other	—	—	—	—	—	—	Few sperm

Contaminants

The urine sediment may contain hair and other fibers, mucous threads, spermatozoa, starch granules, and oil globules, which should be disregarded.

Fat

Fat is excreted in the urine in increased amounts in patients with the nephrotic syndrome and may appear in three forms: free fat droplets, oval fat bodies, which are tubular epithelial cells filled with fat and fatty casts. Polarized light will often show cholesterol crystals within the fat as Maltese cross-shaped light patterns.

Suggested Readings

Abuelo JG. The diagnosis of hematuria. Arch Intern Med 1983;143:967–970.
Abuelo JG. Proteinuria. Ann Intern Med 1983;98:186–191.
Chavers BM, Vernier RL. Proteinuria and enzymuria. Semin Nephrol 1986;6:371–388.
Graff L. A handbook of routine urinalysis. Philadelphia: J.B. Lippincott Co, 1983.
Kiel DP, Moskowitz MA. The urinalysis: A critical appraisal. Med Clin NA 1987;71:607–625.

URINALYSIS PROBLEMS

Answer the following questions after looking at urinalysis results given on Table 11.1.

1. A 40-year-old woman is sent to you for a second opinion. She has had painless gross hematuria for 3 days. An IVP looking for urinary stones or a renal tumor was normal. She feels otherwise well. Scr is normal. The patient's urologist recommended that she undergo cystoscopy to eliminate the possibility of a bleeding tumor of the bladder.
   A. Should she undergo this cystoscopy? Why?
   B. What diagnosis do you suspect?
2. A 5-year-old child has short stature. Some preliminary studies show normal BUN, Scr and blood glucose concentration. Serum electrolyte levels in mEq/L are Na^+ 140, Cl^- 111, K^+ 3.3, HCO_3^- 17, gap 12, and arterial pH = 7.31. What is the most likely diagnosis?
3. A 20-year-old male track star comes to your office in the afternoon

after having voided red-brown urine. He had just run a marathon that morning. Would you evaluate the patient for hematuria? Why?

4. A 40-year-old man with a bleeding gastric ulcer one year earlier is admitted with a history of passing maroon-colored bloody stool for one day. One week before his Scr and BUN were 0.9 and 10 mg/dl. His pulse is 130/min and his BP is 60–70/30 mm Hg; it remains in this range despite transfusion because of continued gastrointestinal bleeding as revealed by blood continually suctioned from a naso-gastric tube. Urine output via a Foley catheter is only 20 cc/hour. Scr is 2.2 (normal<1.5 mg/dl) and BUN is 48 mg/dl (normal<20 mg/dl). What is the most likely cause of the elevated BUN and creatinine?

5. A 30-year-old woman comes to your office complaining of a dry mouth and waking up at night to urinate. What is the most likely diagnosis?

6. A 22-year-old previously healthy woman has had fever (temperature is 104°F), right-sided flank pain for 24 hours. The intern's diagnosis is acute pyelonephritis. Is this a reasonable diagnosis?

7. A 22-year-old medical student goes jogging before school as part of an effort to lose weight. He has reduced his food intake by skipping breakfast and supper. His first class was a laboratory where the student performed a urinalysis on his own urine. What is your advice to the student?

chapter 12

Hypertension

Rex L. Mahnensmith

Chronic hypertension is a major health problem for industrialized societies and is a common clinical challenge for the practicing physician. In the United States the incidence of hypertension is 20–25% among all individuals over the age of 35 years and increases with age to 35–40% among patients 60 years or older. Hypertension is the predominant risk factor for premature cardiac and cerebrovascular disease. From large population studies, it is clear that the frequency of stroke, heart failure and myocardial infarction is directly related to the height of the blood pressure: the higher the pressure, the higher the rate of morbidity and mortality. Yet, the greatest overall toll on health occurs among those individuals with only minimally elevated blood pressure, simply because this group is so much larger than those with more severe hypertension. The ultimate importance in recognizing and understanding hypertension is that it is treatable—and treatment makes a difference. Just as the risk of disability and death increases as the severity of hypertension worsens, so does it diminish as treatment lowers the blood pressure. Thus, recognition of hypertension in an individual allows the physician to predict future risk of cardiovascular disease and to intervene in a preventive manner. Beyond recognizing hypertensive individuals and educating them about its complications, the management challenge to the physician is to prescribe effective therapy with the least side effect. Understanding the various factors interacting in the pathogenesis of hypertension is a prerequisite to success in this clinical endeavor.

Definition

In common medical parlance, "hypertension" denotes a chronic elevation of the systemic arterial blood pressure. It would be more explicit to use the term "systemic arterial hypertension," so as to convey proper meaning and distinction from other medical conditions such as "pulmonary hypertension" (elevated pressure in the pulmonary arteries) and "portal hypertension" (elevated pressure in the portal veins). "Benign hypertension" is a time-honored designation, implying systemic arterial hypertension without apparent complications. This term is misapplied, since apparently benign hypertension often leads to untoward complications. It really should be discarded. This is contrasted to "malignant hypertension," which connotes severe hypertension with rapidly progressive life-threatening complications and is a medical emergency.

A wide range of blood pressures exists among healthy individuals with no natural demarcation between "normal" values and "elevated" values. Also, in healthy individuals blood pressure rises steadily from early childhood through the late adolescent years and naturally fluctuates throughout the day, sometimes by as much as 50/20 mm Hg. Thus, a strict physiologic definition of when blood pressures are elevated and constitute hypertension is not possible. Nevertheless, it is clear that arterial blood pressure is normally regulated within a range that provides adequate tissue perfusion with minimal vascular and organ trauma.

Accordingly, an operational concept has evolved from population studies which define **hypertension** as that level of sustained systemic arterial pressure which results over time in end-organ damage, most commonly in the eyes, the brain, the heart, the kidneys and the vasculature. An essential corollary is that effective antihypertensive therapy, if prescribed early, will prevent these end-organ complications.

This definition is somewhat problematic because the incidence of cardiovascular complications rises, even as average blood pressures exceed 110/70 mm Hg. Nevertheless, most authorities agree that blood pressures consistently greater than 140/90 mm Hg are undesirably high, because there is no doubt that premature cardiovascular morbid-

Table 12.1.
Clinical Classification of Blood Pressure[a]

	Blood Pressure (mm Hg)	Category
Diastolic	<85	Normal
	85–89	High normal
	90–104	Mild hypertension
	105–114	Moderate hypertension
	≥115	Severe hypertension
Systolic[b]	<140	Normal
	140–159	Borderline isolated systolic hypertension
	≥160	Isolated systolic hypertension

[a] Modified from The 1988 Report of the Joint National Committee on Detection, Evaluation and Treatment of High Blood Pressure. Arch Int Med 148:1023–1038, 1988.
[b] When diastolic blood pressure <90 mm Hg.

ity is associated with this blood pressure and therapeutic intervention at this level reduces the incidence and risk of complications.[a]

The diastolic blood pressure has been the traditional focus in gauging severity. Accordingly, sustained diastolic pressures between 90 and 104 mm Hg are classified as mild hypertension; diastolic pressures between 105 and 114 mm Hg are categorized as moderate hypertension; and diastolic pressures greater than 114 mm Hg are classified as severe hypertension (Table 12.1).

Isolated systolic hypertension is an additional concept defined as sustained systolic blood pressures greater than 160 mm Hg with diastolic values less than 90 mm Hg. Isolated systolic hypertension results from atherosclerotic loss of elasticity of the arterial tree and is mainly a problem in the elderly. Cardiovascular morbidity and mortality rise significantly with incremental isolated systolic elevations in a manner similar to that seen with diastolic elevations.

These definitions pertain only to nonpregnant adults. Ambient blood pressures in healthy children and pregnant women are typically lower.

---

[a]The World Health Organization has defined hypertension as systolic pressures greater than 160 mm Hg and diastolic pressures greater than 95 mm Hg. While these criteria have gained worldwide acceptance, the Joint National Committee on Detection, Evaluation and Treatment of High Blood Pressure, sponsored by the National Institutes of Health has modified these limits downward to 140/90 mm Hg.

Table 12.2
Hypertension in Children and Adolescents

Age (years)	Upper Limit of Normal Blood Pressure (mm Hg)
<6	115/75
6–9	120/80
10–12	125/82
13–18	135/85

For children below the age of 6 years, 115/75 mm Hg is the upper limit of normal; for children ages 6 to 9, values greater than 120/80 mm Hg are hypertensive; for youths ages 10–12, 125/82 mm Hg is the upper limit of normal; and for adolescents ages 13–18, values greater than 135/85 mm Hg are hypertensive (Table 12.2). During pregnancy, blood pressure is normally low during the first and second trimesters and returns toward the nonpregnant values during the third trimester. Blood pressure values which rise more than 30/15 mm Hg during the course of pregnancy or exceed 140/90 mm Hg are hypertensive and are associated with maternal and fetal complications.

Etiology

The vast majority (90–95%) of adults with documented hypertension do not have an identifiable cause and are, therefore, categorized as having **primary or essential** hypertension. In the remaining 5–10% of hypertensive adults, the hypertension arises as a consequence of a definable disease process and is, therefore, designated as secondary hypertension.

In children, secondary hypertension is probably responsible for a greater proportion of cases than in adults, although reliable data on this question are scarce. In pediatric practice, as in adult practice, hypertension is usually mild (and asymptomatic) and essential (primary) hypertension is the predominant diagnosis. On the other hand, in cases seen in referral centers, the hypertension is usually severe and a majority of these cases have a definable cause. Among these children with secondary hypertension, nearly 80% have a primary renal abnormality; 10–20% have renal artery stenosis or coarctation of the aorta; and the remainder have chiefly endocrine abnormalities such as pheochromocytoma, aldosteronism or congenital adrenal hyperplasia.

Common etiologies of arterial hypertension are listed in Table 12.3.

Table 12.3.
Principal Causes of Hypertension

I. Idiopathic (essential, primary)
II. Renal
    A. Renovascular stenosis
      1. Fibromuscular dysplasia
      2. Atherosclerotic
    B. Renal parenchymal disease
    C. Obstructive nephropathy
III. Adrenal
    A. Medullary-pheochromocytoma
    B. Cortical
      1. Primary aldosteronism
        a. Adrenal adenoma
        b. Bilateral adrenal hyperplasia
      2. Cushing's disease
IV. Exogenous agents
    A. Oral contraceptives
    B. Sympathetic amines (decongestants)
    C. Nonsteroidal anti-inflammatory drugs
    D. High dose corticosteroid administration
    E. Disorders simulating mineralocorticoid excess
      1. Licorice
      2. Chewing tobacco
V. Miscellaneous
    A. Coarctation of aorta
    B. Acute stress

Pathogenesis

No matter what the etiology of the hypertensive state, the circulatory physiology is disturbed in all individuals. Before this pathophysiology can be meaningfully discussed, a brief review of normal blood pressure regulation is in order.

Determinants of Normal Blood Pressure

The pressure required to move blood through the arterial network is generated by cardiac contraction and sustained by the resistance to flow offered by the peripheral arteries and arterioles. Accordingly, the cardiac output (CO) and the peripheral vascular resistance (PVR) are the primary determinants of systemic blood pressure. The relationship between the mean arterial pressure (MAP) and its primary determinants is expressed as follows:

$$MAP = CO \times PVR$$

Cardiac output is determined by plasma volume, cardiac stroke volume, heart rate and myocardial contractility. Peripheral vascular resistance is a function of the balance of humoral vasoconstrictor and vasodilator factors, adrenergic activity and intrinsic smooth muscle tone of the arterioles (Fig. 12.1).

Blood pressure is normally regulated above the lowest level that supports vital organ perfusion and below a level that produces organ and vascular damage. Four integrated sensor-effector systems maintain the blood pressure within these limits through feedback modulation of CO and PVR. These are the **arterial baroreceptor reflex,** renal regulation of **plasma volume,** the **renin-angiotensin-aldosterone system** and **vascular autoregulation.**

Arterial Baroreceptor Reflex. Baroreceptors in the aortic arch and carotid arteries sense perfusion pressure and wall tension and signal the brainstem through the afferent autonomic nervous system. The brainstem then modulates efferent adrenergic and vagal activity which in turn governs myocardial contractility, heart rate and PVR. These

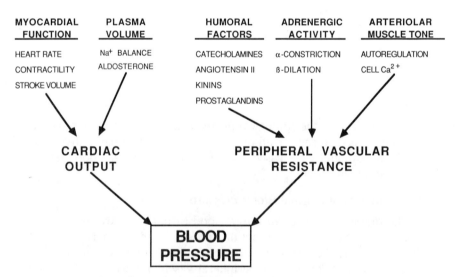

Figure 12.1.   Physiologic determinants of arterial blood pressure.

feedback mechanisms are nearly instantaneous and effect moment to moment governance of arterial pressure. Adrenergic activity also has a more gradual influence on PVR and plasma volume by promoting renal renin production and directly increasing renal tubular Na^+ reabsorption.

Plasma Volume. Renal regulation of Na^+ balance governs plasma Na^+ content, which largely determines plasma volume. A fall in blood pressure promotes renal retention of Na^+, which slowly restores blood pressure through expansion of plasma volume and an increase in CO. Conversely, a rise in blood pressure normally promotes a diuresis, thereby lowering blood pressure through a contraction of plasma volume and a decline in CO (see **sodium regulation** in Chapter 1). In these contexts, Na^+ excretion is modulated directly by changes in GFR and glomerular perfusion pressure and indirectly by aldosterone and changes in local prostaglandin, adrenergic and angiotensin activity. Thus, an intricate physiologic integration of renal Na^+ balance and blood pressure control is apparent.

Renin-Angiotensin-Aldosterone System. Following a fall in blood pressure, the kidneys produce renin. This production is mediated through a decline in glomerular perfusion pressure, a decline in the NaCl content of the distal tubular fluid and an increase in local adrenergic activity. Renin itself is not a pressor substance but is an enzyme that catalyzes production of angiotensin I, which is then converted to angiotensin II. Angiotensin II increases blood pressure directly as an arteriolar vasoconstrictor and indirectly as a stimulant of aldosterone production, which in turn promotes renal Na^+ reabsorption. In addition, through differential vasoconstrictive actions on the afferent and efferent glomerular arterioles, angiotensin II raises filtration fraction, which also enhances tubular Na^+ reabsorption (see chapter on **volume disorders**). Finally, angiotensin II directly stimulates tubular Na^+ reabsorption. Thus, this system subserves long-term regulation of blood pressure through changes in both PVR and plasma volume.

Vascular Autoregulation. Arterioles have an intrinsic capability to alter muscular tone in response to local perfusion pressures, termed autoregulation. In particular, when CO rises, arterioles constrict, protecting capillaries and tissues from hyperperfusion. Local arteriolar dilation or constriction thereby modulates tissue perfusion over a range of systemic pressures. This activity participates in setting total PVR and thereby affects blood pressure.

These four systems operate synergistically as modulators of systemic arterial blood pressure. The kidney integrates these operations and stabilizes blood pressure over the long term, complementing the more immediate myocardial and arteriolar responses. For example, a drop in blood pressure will immediately trigger renal Na^+ retention through a fall in GFR and filtered Na^+ and at the same time will activate the renin-angiotensin-aldosterone system, which in turn leads to angiotensin and aldosterone-mediated renal Na^+ retention. Concomitantly, carotid baroreceptor activation will increase adrenergic activity, leading to an adrenergic-mediated increase in tubular Na^+ reabsorption and augmentation of renin-angiotensin-aldosterone production. The resulting rise in plasma volume defends against the initial fall in blood pressure. This central role of the kidney assumes particular importance when we consider the pathophysiologic mechanisms in essential hypertension.

Secondary Hypertension

An analysis of factors responsible for hypertension begins with first principles, namely, the CO and the PVR. When hypertension is secondary to an identifiable disease process, the pathophysiologic mechanisms are readily apparent. For example, with **pheochromocytoma,** i.e. a catecholamine-producing tumor of the adrenal medulla, high circulating epinephrine and norepinephrine concentrations both constrict peripheral blood vessels and heighten CO. An aldosterone-producing **adrenal adenoma** produces hypertension through renal Na^+ retention and associated plasma volume expansion. With unilateral **renal artery stenosis,** e.g. from fibromuscular dysplasia or atherosclerosis, renin output from the underperfused kidney causes angiotensin II-mediated vasoconstriction and aldosterone-induced renal Na^+ retention, while **renal parenchymal disease** impairs Na^+ excretion, expanding plasma volume and increasing CO. In **Cushing's syndrome,** i.e. excessive cortisol production, hypertension results from the high levels of cortisol, which causes Na^+ retention through its weak mineralocorticoid action and increases production of renin substrate, thereby increasing angiotensin II and aldosterone. Hypertension associated with **oral contraceptive** use also arises from an increase in renin substrate production plus the mild Na^+-retaining effect of estrogen. The mechanisms of hypertension in **coarctation of the aorta** are uncertain. In many patients renal blood flow is reduced because of the fibrous aortic stricture characteristic of this disease. Thus, renin, angiotensin and aldosterone participate as mediators, causing a combina-

Table 12.4.
Pathogenetic Mechanisms in Secondary Hypertension

Disorder	Mediators	Pathophysiologic Mechanisms
Pheochromocytoma	↑ Catecholamines	Vasoconstriction
		↑ Cardiac output
Primary aldosteronism	↑ Aldosterone	Na$^+$ retention
Renal artery stenosis	↑ Renin^a	Vasoconstriction
	↑ Aldosterone	Na$^+$ retention
Renal insufficiency	↓ GFR	Na$^+$ retention
	↑ Renin^a	Vasoconstriction
Cushing's syndrome	↑ Cortisol	Na$^+$ retention
	↑ Renin substrate	Vasoconstriction
Oral contraceptives	↑ Renin substrate	Vasoconstriction
	Estrogen	Na$^+$ retention
Aortic coarctation	↑ Renin	Vasoconstriction
	↑ Aldosterone	Na$^+$ retention

^{a}A minority of cases.

tion of peripheral vasoconstriction and renal Na$^+$ retention (Table 12.4).

Primary (Essential) Hypertension

In individuals with essential hypertension, the mechanisms for generating and maintaining elevated blood pressure are less well-defined than for secondary hypertension. Several disturbances in the physiologic control mechanisms are apparent, exhibiting variably important roles in different individuals. However, no single pathophysiologic process by itself consistently accounts for the rise in systemic arterial pressure.

The hemodynamic hallmark of essential hypertension is an increase in PVR. Cardiac output is usually normal, although there is a subset of younger individuals with hypertension with a "hyperkinetic circulation," which is characterized by elevated heart rate and CO. Plasma volume is variable among individuals with essential hypertension: in most untreated patients, plasma volume is slightly contracted, exhibiting an inverse relation to the height of the arterial pressure; however, owing to an impairment in Na$^+$ excretion, it remains inappropriately high for the level of diastolic pressure. In blacks and obese persons, plasma volume tends to be increased and tends to vary with salt intake, leading to salt-sensitive hypertension. Nevertheless, in these latter persons, an increased PVR is evident and is largely responsible for the elevated blood pressure.

The sustained increase in PVR and inappropriate Na^+ retention in essential hypertension arise through several mechanisms. These include:

1) Increased adrenergic activity
2) Increased circulating angiotensin II
3) Atherosclerotic arteriolar narrowing
4) Impaired pressure-natriuresis
5) A natriuretic hormone

Increased Adrenergic Activity. Heightened adrenergic activity is at least partially responsible for the increased PVR of essential hypertension.

> Evidence for this includes the following:
>
> a) An elevation in arterial pressure should reflexly reduce adrenergic activity, but most hypertensive individuals have either normal or increased circulating norepinephrine and epinephrine levels, indicating a resetting of the baroreceptor feedback;
>
> b) A hyperadrenergic state often characterizes early hypertension in young adults;
>
> c) Pharmacologic agents which inhibit adrenergic activity either centrally or peripherally will lower the blood pressure of many hypertensive patients;
>
> d) Normotensive blood relatives of individuals with essential hypertension exhibit exaggerated adrenergic responses to various stresses;
>
> e) Animals with spontaneous hypertension consistently feature an inappropriately active adrenergic nervous system.

Factors involved in the genesis of the enhanced adrenergic state in essential hypertension are unknown. Chronic stress may contribute. However, how increased adrenergic activity maintains the hypertensive state is known. As depicted in Figure 12.2, both the CO and PVR are increased through direct myocardial and arteriolar actions. More important, however, are the renal consequences: renal adrenergic activity directly enhances tubular Na^+ reabsorption and activates the renin-angiotensin-aldosterone system which further augments renal Na^+ retention and peripheral vasoconstriction. Thus, the expected

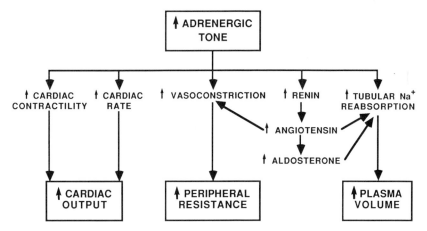

Figure 12.2. Cardiovascular and renal consequences of increased adrenergic tone. Modified from Rose BD. Pathogenesis of essential hypertension. In: Rose BD. Pathophysiology of renal disease. New York: McGraw-Hill Book Co., 1987:469–496.

natriuresis that should follow an elevation in CO is thwarted and hypertension is sustained.

Increased Circulating Angiotensin II. Approximately 70% of individuals with essential hypertension have either normal or elevated plasma renin levels. As with adrenergic activity, even normal renin activity can be considered physiologically inappropriate, since elevations in blood pressure should suppress renin secretion. As explained above, it is likely that the inappropriately high renin activity is partly a consequence of increased adrenergic activity. In longstanding hypertension with nephrosclerosis, renal arteriosclerosis and vascular narrowing cause local ischemia, which additionally stimulates renin production. The resultant increase in circulating angiotensin II sustains hypertension through two mechanisms: 1) direct peripheral vascular constriction and 2) renal Na^+ retention through preglomerular vasoconstriction, a direct effect on the renal tubule and stimulation of aldosterone output (Fig. 12.3).

Atherosclerotic Arteriolar Narrowing. With prolonged systemic hypertension, functional and reversible arteriolar constriction gives way to fixed anatomic thickening of the arteriolar wall, resulting in irreversible narrowing of arteriolar lumina. These changes feature

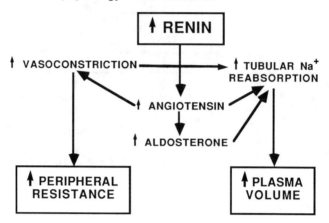

Figure 12.3. Pathogenetic role of the renin-angiotensin-aldosterone system in essential hypertension.

smooth muscle hypertrophy, fibroblast proliferation and cholesterol accumulation. The pathophysiologic consequence is a fixed increased in PVR. These changes occur throughout all vascular beds but are particularly problematic in the brain, the heart and the kidney, where tissue ischemia and impaired autoregulation result.

Arterial Pressure-Natriuresis Relationship. Increased adrenergic activity and circulating angiotensin II, together with later development of fixed arteriolar narrowing, clearly increase PVR but additionally cause renal Na$^+$ retention and a tendency to plasma volume expansion (Fig. 12.4A). Paradoxically, most individuals with essential hypertension actually have **normal or reduced** plasma volume, producing **normal** CO. This is explained by two phenomena, **pressure-natriuresis** and **natriuretic hormone,** both of which promote Na$^+$ excretion in the hypertensive patient.

When systemic arterial pressure rises, the normal kidney responds with a prompt increase in Na$^+$ excretion, causing a proportionate contraction of plasma volume and return of blood pressure to normal (Fig. 12.5). In individuals with essential hypertension, this mechanism often reduces plasma volume to or below normal, despite the Na$^+$ retaining actions of the adrenergic and renin-angiotensin-aldosterone systems (Fig. 12.4B).

Impaired Pressure-Natriuresis. For hypertension to be sustained this pressure-natriuresis relationship must be impaired. Were it intact,

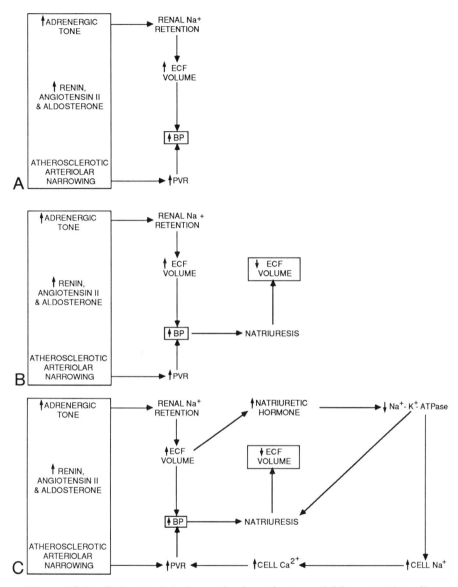

Figure 12.4. Pathophysiologic mechanisms in essential hypertension. A) Increased adrenergic tone, increased renin and atherosclerotic arteriolar narrowing increase PVR and cause renal Na^+ retention. Extracellular fluid volume expands and blood pressure rises. B) Elevated blood pressure promotes pressure-natriuresis, reducing extracellular volume, but persistent activity of the adrenergic and renin-angiotensin-aldosterone systems blunts the natriuresis and prevents blood pressure normalization. C) Natriuretic hormone is produced. Inhibition of Na^+-K^+-ATPase aids natriuresis, but promotes further peripheral vasoconstriction. Hence, ECF volume is contracted, although not sufficiently to normalize blood pressure, and increased PVR sustains the hypertension.

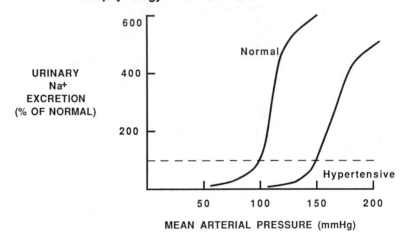

Figure 12.5. Relation between systemic arterial pressure and urinary Na$^+$ excretion in normal and hypertensive individuals. An increase in arterial pressure normally produces a natriuresis sufficient to stabilize the blood pressure and prevent further rise. In hypertensive individuals, the natriuresis response is shifted to the right. Homeostatic Na$^+$ balance *(dashed line)* is achieved only at high arterial pressures, and further pressure-natriuretic responses exhibit a slower rise. Adapted from Guyton AC. Long term regulation of mean arterial pressure: the renal-body fluid pressure control system. In: Guyton AC, ed. Textbook of medical physiology. Philadelphia: W.B. Saunders Co., 1981:259–273.

hypertension would not be possible because correction of any elevation in systemic arterial pressure through natriuresis should occur. In hypertensive individuals, the pressure-natriuresis relationship is shifted to the right (Fig. 12.5). Homeostatic balance between Na$^+$ intake and output is achieved only at the expense of higher systemic arterial pressure. Indeed, if mean arterial pressure were to suddenly decline in a hypertensive individual, as would occur with vasodilator antihypertensive therapy, avid Na$^+$ retention might follow with an attendant rise in the blood pressure towards the preexisting level.

Alteration of the pressure-natriuresis relationship in hypertensive individuals is believed to result from heightened adrenergic and angiotensin II activity within the kidney. This not only increases tubular Na$^+$ transport directly, but also alters periglomerular hemodynamics in such a way as to increase filtration fraction and favor Na$^+$ reabsorption (see Chapter 2 on **volume disorders**). Accordingly, natriuresis sufficient to correct elevated blood pressure is thwarted and the blood pressure remains at hypertensive levels.

Natriuretic Hormone. A consequence of this inappropriate Na^+ retention is the production and secretion of a circulating natriuretic hormone[b] which inhibits plasma membrane Na^+-K^+-ATPase transporters. In the kidney, inhibition of the renal tubular Na^+-K^+-ATPase causes a reduction in renal Na^+ reabsorption, promoting Na^+ excretion and correcting hypervolemia (Fig. 12.6A). In arteriolar smooth muscle, inhibition of Na^+-K^+-ATPase reduces active Na^+ extrusion from the cells, raising cell Na^+ concentration and diminishing passive Na^+ entry. This reduces Ca^{2+} efflux from the cell, which normally occurs through coupled Na^+-Ca^{2+} exchange. The resultant rise in cell Ca^{2+} concentration promotes arteriolar smooth muscle contraction and increases PVR (Fig. 12.4C; 12.6B). Hence, even as plasma volume contracts, hypertension is sustained by heightened vasoconstriction. Indeed, in the majority of untreated individuals with essential hypertension, intracellular Na^+ concentration is high; intracellular Ca^{2+} concentration is high; a circulating inhibitor of plasma membrane Na^+-K^+-ATPase is present; and plasma volume is slightly contracted, although it remains inappropriately high for the level of diastolic blood pressure.

In summary, essential hypertension evolves because hemodynamic regulatory mechanisms are disturbed. As the long-term stabilizer of blood pressure, the kidney assumes a central pathogenetic role. Indeed, the inability of the kidney to appropriately excrete Na^+, except at higher than normal arterial pressure, is held as a primary pathophysiologic defect. This results from persistent intrarenal influences of angiotensin II, aldosterone and adrenergic activity. The resultant production of a natriuretic hormone seems insufficient and maladaptive: renal excretion of Na^+ is promoted and plasma volume is lowered, but the natriuresis remains insufficient to normalize blood pressure. Furthermore, peripheral vascular constriction is heightened. Hence,

---

[b]Two distinct natriuretic hormones have so far been identified. The first is a peptide known as atrial natriuretic factor, which has vasorelaxant properties (see **sodium regulation** in chapter 1). Its role in the pathogenesis of essential hypertension is controversial. The second hormone behaves as a glycoside and is believed to derive from the AV3V region of the hypothalamus. It inhibits plasma membrane Na^+-K^+ ATPase and is believed to participate in the pathogenesis of hypertension, as discussed.

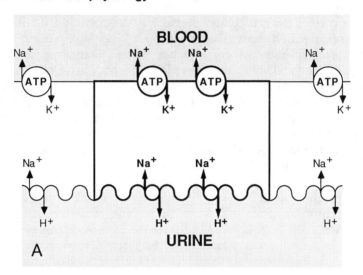

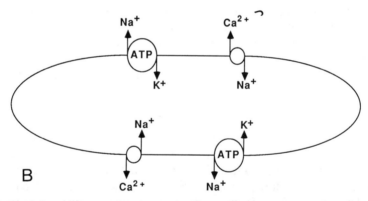

Figure 12.6. Action of plasma membrane Na^+-K^+-ATPase in the renal tubule and arteriolar smooth muscle. A) In the renal tubule, the Na^+-K^+-ATPase pump is located only on the peritubular cell membrane. It catalyzes active extrusion of Na^+ from the cell, generating an inward Na^+ gradient for passive Na^+ transport from the urine across the luminal brush border membrane. Accordingly, transepithelial Na^+ reabsorption is driven by the activity of Na^+-K^+-ATPase. Inhibition of renal Na^+-K^+-ATPase will, therefore, diminish renal tubular Na^+ reabsorption. B) In arteriolar smooth muscle, primary active extrusion of Na^+ via the Na^+-K^+-ATPase pump generates an inward Na^+ gradient. Passive inward movement of Na^+ is coupled to outward Ca^{2+} extrusion. This action helps to maintain a very low cytoplasmic Ca^{2+} content. Inhibition of Na^+-K^+-ATPase will increase cytoplasmic Ca^{2+}, stimulating smooth muscle contraction.

causes and consequences seem caught in a reinforcing cycle and the kidney stands central in its failure to provide complete regulatory correction (Fig. 12.4C).

Clinical Features

Manifestations of Uncomplicated Hypertension

Young individuals who are destined to develop sustained hypertension often have blood pressures higher than their peers, although still within the accepted "normal" range. Their blood pressures tend to rise steadily over many years and typically reach a level that requires therapy between the ages of 30 and 50. Most hypertensive patients remain asymptomatic even after many years. Thus, hypertension is discovered most often by chance during physical examinations for other purposes. This is unfortunate, for too often hypertension is first detected only after vital organ injury causes specific symptoms, such as those from a stroke or myocardial infarction.

Symptoms that can be directly attributable to elevated arterial pressure, headache and lightheadedness are present in less than 25% of hypertensive patients. Because the early years of evolving hypertension are characterized by fluctuations in the arterial pressure, these symptoms, if they occur, are typically infrequent and fleeting and do not arouse suspicion. As hypertension becomes more sustained, these symptoms become more frequent and noticeable, especially when elevations are severe (diastolic blood pressure >115 mm Hg). However, some patients are asymptomatic with diastolic blood pressure above 115 mm Hg and rarely even above 140–150 mm Hg!

The physical examination in uncomplicated hypertension is usually unremarkable other than the elevated blood pressure reading, unless one is dealing with secondary hypertension (see below).

Complications of Hypertension

Whether primary or secondary in etiology, years of uncontrolled hypertension may produce damage in several vital structures, particularly the eyes, brain, heart, kidneys and aorta (Table 12.5). The likelihood of organ injury mounts with the duration and aorta (Table 12.5). The likelihood of organ injury mounts with the duration and severity of the blood pressure elevation.

Eyes. Patients with "benign" hypertension develop atherosclerotic

Table 12.5.
Complications of Established Hypertension

Eye	Brain	Heart	Kidney	Aorta
Retinal ischemia	Transient ischemia	Hypertrophy	Glomerulosclerosis	Accelerated atherosclerosis
Retinal hemorrhage	Lacunar infarction	Ventricular failure	Proteinuria	Aortic aneurysm
Papilledema	Thrombotic infarction	Angina	Progressive insufficiency	Aortic dissection
	Hemorrhage	Infarction	Uremia	Occlusion of branches

thickening of the walls of the retinal arterioles that can be seen on fun-duscopy. This is manifest as arteriolar narrowing and arteriovenous nicking, in which the thickened arterioles nick or compress the retinal veins at crossover points. Loss of normal transparency of the vessel wall may produce a widened reflectance of the examining light from the arterioles and opacification of the wall obscures the red color of the blood, resulting in "copper or silver wiring." Fortunately these changes rarely cause visual impairment.

Other eye complications may cause blurred vision. Occasionally, vessels will rupture under pressure, leaving a small flame-shaped hemorrhage, or they may completely occlude, producing a small pale infarct. Healed hemorrhages or infarcts will appear as exudates or cotton wool spots. These changes usually indicate severe hypertension.

Brain. Deep in the brain, small arteries and arterioles undergo stenosing intimal thickening with poststenotic microaneurysm formation. These vessels may hemorrhage or occlude, producing a stroke syndrome or neurologic deficit unique to the involved region of brain.

Heart. Longstanding hypertension predisposes the coronary arteries to atherosclerosis and increases the incidence of angina pectoris and myocardial infarction. Also, high peripheral vascular resistance chronically increases afterload on the left ventricle, which results in left ventricular hypertrophy. The patient might complain of dyspnea on exertion, easy fatigability or palpitations. Physical examination may reveal increased force and lateral displacement of the cardiac apical impulse or a fourth heart sound. Left ventricular hypertrophy may be detected early in its evolution by echocardiography or electrocardiography and only later becomes manifest on chest X-ray. Decompensation of the left ventricle may be triggered by acute ischemia or a further rise in blood pressure or might slowly evolve, resulting in signs and symptoms of overt left-sided congestive heart failure.

Kidneys. Longstanding hypertension induces both vascular and glomerular damage in the kidney. Typically, larger intrarenal vessels show fibrous atherosclerotic thickening of the intima with narrowing of the lumen. Smaller arteries exhibit similar changes as well as smooth muscle hypertrophy and layered proliferation. In the afferent glomerular arterioles a gradual eosinophilic hyaline thickening evolves, a consequence of fracturing damage and the deposition of proteins into the arteriolar wall. These changes impair the kidney's ability to autoregulate renal blood flow and can result in prerenal azotemia and excessive Na^+ retention when arterial pressure is lowered, even down to a high-normal range.

Glomerular damage evolves from glomerular hypertension and chronic ischemia. Initially, injury produces sclerotic shrinkage of a single capillary tuft in a few scattered glomeruli. Eventually, sclerosis generalizes within a glomerulus, leaving a small eosinophilic, scarred glomerular remnant. As earlier affected glomeruli undergo this process, blood flow is diverted and perfusion pressures rise in less-affected glomeruli. Higher pressures within these glomeruli accelerates their injury. Collectively, these vascular and glomerular changes are known as **benign arteriolar nephrosclerosis.**

Mild proteinuria is the usual clinical manifestation of benign arteriolar nephrosclerosis and correlates with duration and severity of the hypertension. Gradual loss of GFR usually accompanies proteinuria with slow progression to ESRD in a small number of cases. Mild hypertension usually causes no appreciable impairment in renal function.

Aorta. Large vessel atherosclerosis is accelerated with hypertension and results more from the denuding stresses of pounding blood flow than from the simple sustained elevation in the mean arterial pressure per se. Aortic aneurysm formation and intramural dissection are consequences of this and are seen most frequently in the distal thoracic or abdominal regions. Aneurysms enlarge slowly and are often asymptomatic, until they leak or are about to rupture. Intramural dissection is always a painful crisis and is usually accompanied by signs of vascular occlusion and shock.

Secondary Hypertension

Additional clinical manifestations specific to the underlying cause may be seen in the secondary forms of hypertension.

Renal Parenchymal Disease. Hypertension due to primary renal parenchymal disease is accompanied by an abnormal urinalysis and an elevated BUN and Scr.

Renovascular Stenosis. This often has features substantially different from essential hypertension. These include: 1) onset of hypertension in an individual younger than 20 or older than 50 years of age; 2) an abrupt rise in blood pressure over a previously stable baseline; 3) severe hypertension with funduscopic changes; 4) an abdominal or flank bruit; 5) renal insufficiency without urinary sediment abnormalities (suggests bilateral renal artery stenosis).

Two clinical scenarios are highly suggestive of renal artery stenosis with renovascular hypertension: a) the sudden onset of moderate-to-severe hypertension in a young woman with an abdominal bruit and no family history of hypertension is a classic presentation for renal artery fibromuscular dysplasia; and b) a sudden rise in arterial pressure above previously controlled levels in an already hypertensive elderly individual suggests the evolution of an atherosclerotic renal artery stenosis.

Pheochromocytoma. This is a rare cause of hypertension that can have very distinctive features. One should suspect pheochromocytoma when there are **paroxysmal** elevations of blood pressure with head **pain,** cardiac **palpitations, pallor** and **perspiration** (the five **P's**), accelerated or refractory hypertension and hypermetabolism with weight loss. These symptoms reflect periodic release of catecholamines from the adrenal medullary tumor. While these intermittent phenomena are uniquely suggestive of the diagnosis, roughly 50% of these patients will have sustained elevations of arterial pressure with minimal paroxysmal adrenergic symptoms.

Primary Aldosteronism. Hypertension with hypokalemia from urinary K^+ wasting suggests primary aldosterone excess, arising from a solitary adrenal adenoma or bilateral adrenal hyperplasia. Edema hardly ever accompanies primary aldosteronism, because the kidney ordinarily "escapes" the Na^+ retentive action of aldosterone. Metabolic alkalosis usually accompanies the hypokalemia and mild hypernatremia occurs occasionally. One must distinguish this cause of hypokalemia from the secondary hyperaldosteronism of renal artery stenosis and from diuretic therapy.

Cushing's Syndrome. This arises from glucocorticoid excess. It presents with easily recognizable physical features: a rounded face with fleshy cheeks, fine textured hair on the face and trunk, truncal obesity and ecchymoses. Muscle atrophy from protein catabolism results in thinning of the limbs. Biochemical abnormalities include hypokalemia and metabolic alkalosis (a mineralocorticoid effect) and elevated glucose (a glucocorticoid effect). If the syndrome results from a pituitary adenoma, headache or visual field cuts may dominate other symptoms. Adrenal cortical adenomas themselves do not usually cause local symptoms.

Coarctation of the Aorta. Coarctation is usually asymptomatic aside from the manifestations of hypertension itself. On physical examination the pressure drop across the stenosis produces blood pressure differences between the two arms or between the arms and the legs.

Accelerated Hypertension-Malignant Hypertension

Accelerated hypertension refers to a rapid elevation in arterial pressure, regardless of etiology. Diastolic pressures are usually in excess of 130 mm Hg. **Malignant hypertension** is a clinical syndrome of overt end-organ damage arising from a rapidly progressive elevation in blood pressure. Intense vasospasm is present, with endothelial damage and fibrinoid necrosis in the arterioles of many organs, particularly the eye, the brain and the kidney. Organ damage develops from ischemia resulting from the intense vasospasm and hyperperfusion injury.

Eyes. Very high pressure in the delicate retinal vessels causes reflex vasospasm and flame-shaped hemorrhages. Edema of the optic nerve head, known as papilledema, is usually seen in malignant hypertension. With such severe retinopathy, visual blurring is usually present.

Brain. In the brain, the clinical manifestations reflect the intense small vessel vasospasm and focal tissue ischemia. Over time, the tightly spastic vessels yield to the rapidly rising pressures, allowing hyperperfusion damage and leakage of plasma into the perivascular tissue. Cerebral edema and the clinical syndrome of hypertensive encephalopathy result, manifested by headache, agitation, lethargy, confusion, stupor and coma. Focal neurologic deficits may appear.

Kidneys. In the kidneys intimal thickening and fibrinoid necrosis of the arteriolar wall markedly narrow small arteriolar lumena, a development known as **malignant arteriolar nephrosclerosis.** The glomeruli become acutely ischemic and progressive renal failure ensues. Proteinuria, hematuria and granular casts are usual, and together with renal failure present a nephritic picture!

Heart. The rising PVR presents an increasing afterload to the left ventricle, resulting in left-sided heart failure with pulmonary venous congestion and pulmonary edema. Myocardial ischemia is also common from the high work load, wall tension and myocardial oxygen demands.

Diagnosis

Initial Evaluation

Blood pressure fluctuates widely throughout the day. Both systolic and diastolic pressure change with rest, exercise, excitement, sleep and the multiple stresses common in everyday life. Therefore, multiple determinations of blood pressure should be obtained over time in order to characterize an average level and to document a trend, particularly when the levels are high normal or only mildly elevated.

Once hypertension is identified, the diagnostic evaluation has three purposes: 1) to differentiate primary hypertension from secondary hypertension; 2) to delineate risk factors which might accelerate cardiovascular disease; and 3) to assess vital organ damage.

Every patient must have a complete history and physical examination. While 90–95% of adults with elevated blood pressure have essential hypertension (Table 12.6), it is prudent to look carefully for symp-

Table 12.6.
Relative Incidence of Major
Causes of Hypertension in Adults

Essential hypertension	90–95%
Renal parenchymal disease	4–5%
Renovascular disease	2–5%
Mineralocorticoid excess	<1%
Pheochromocytoma	<1%
Cushing's syndrome	<1%
Oral contraceptives	<1%
Coarctation of aorta	<1%

Table 12.7.
Minimum Evaluation of the Hypertensive Individual

Complete history and physical examination
Serum creatinine, K^+ and Ca^{2+} concentrations
Blood glucose, cholesterol, uric acid and triglyceride concentrations
Hemoglobin, hematocrit
Urinalysis: macro- and microscopic
Electrocardiogram

---

toms or signs typical of some secondary cause. This is especially important among children and adolescents with severe or symptomatic hypertension, who are likely to have a secondary etiology for their elevated blood pressure. A minimum laboratory evaluation to screen for secondary causes and to assess important risk factors should include serum creatinine, Ca^{2+}, K^+, glucose, cholesterol and triglyceride concentrations, complete blood count, urinalysis, chest X-ray and electrocardiogram. Should a secondary cause be suggested, then further specific testing is warranted.

Renal Parenchymal Disease

The most common secondary cause of hypertension is renal parenchymal disease. The history, physical examination and general laboratory evaluation will identify almost all of these patients.

Renovascular Hypertension

Once the possibility of renovascular hypertension is entertained, renal angiography with bilateral renal vein renin sampling is the diagnostic test of choice. Arteriography localizes a stenosis and assesses its severity; only stenoses greater than 70% will compromise perfusion and cause elevation of renin output. Thus, renal vein renin sampling must be performed to assess pathophysiologic significance of a demonstrated renal artery stenosis. If the stenosis is responsible for the hypertension, the renal vein on the affected side usually has elevated renin activity while renin output from the other kidney is usually suppressed by the transmitted arterial hypertension.

Primary Aldosteronism

Spontaneous hypokalemia suggests primary hyperaldosteronism, but hypokalemia in a patient receiving a diuretic has little meaning unless severe. The diagnosis is made by documenting elevated plasma or urine aldosterone levels as well as suppressed plasma renin activity, which occurs because of feedback inhibition of renin secretion by the aldosterone-induced hypervolemia. Once hyperaldosteronism is diagnosed chemically, the physician must employ adrenal CAT scanning to distinguish an adrenal adenoma from bilateral adrenal hyperplasia.

Cushing's Syndrome

Cushing's syndrome is less difficult to diagnose than primary aldosteronism because of the characteristic physical changes induced by the glucocorticoid excess. Diagnosis requires demonstration of autonomous and excessive cortisol production.

Most cases are identified by an early morning elevation in the concentration of plasma cortisol after administration of an overnight suppressive dose of dexamethasone (1 mg at 10 PM), which normally turns off all endogenous production of cortisol. Confirmation requires documentation of elevated urinary free cortisol and 17-hydroxycorticosteroid excretion over a 24-hour period during continuous suppression with oral dexamethasone administration. Then, the physician must distinguish a pituitary adenoma with overproduction of ACTH as the cause of hypercortisolism from an adrenal adenoma with autonomous overproduction of cortisol, which suppresses ACTH.

Pheochromocytoma

Pheochromocytoma is diagnosed by documentation of excessive urinary catecholamine and metabolite excretion (metanephrine and vanillyllmandelic acid) in a 24-hour urine sample. If performed properly, assaying plasma levels of norepinephrine and epinephrine before and after administration of clonidine is probably more sensitive as a diagnostic test. Plasma catecholamines are suppressed by oral clonidine in normal people but not in those with pheochromocytoma. Abdominal CAT scanning usually visualizes the adrenal medullary adenoma.

Coarctation of the Aorta

In coarctation of the aorta the diagnosis can be made through the history and the physical examination. All patients below the age of 30 with hypertension should have blood pressures measured in both arms and one leg at least once to assess for this condition. Combined with a delay in the pulses ("radial-femoral lag"), the certainty of diagnosis approaches 100% when there is a substantial differential in the blood pressures in the arms (normally, the left arm is up to 10 mm Hg higher than the right arm) or when (right) arm pressure is greater than leg pressure. Aortography confirms the diagnosis.

Treatment

The goal of any therapeutic program is to lower the blood pressure into the normal range (<140/90 mm Hg). Such treatment reduces the excess morbidity and mortality from the long-term complications of hypertension.

Nonpharmacologic therapy should always be applied and initially can be used alone if the blood pressure is only mildly elevated. This includes dietary Na^+ restriction, weight reduction in obese individuals, cessation of smoking, moderation of alcohol use and daily aerobic activity. Specific pharmacologic therapy should be added if nonpharmacologic maneuvers do not lower the blood pressure satisfactorily or if there is evidence of end-organ harm. The antihypertensive drugs fall into five classes: diuretics, adrenergic inhibitors, direct vasodilators, angiotensin-converting enzyme inhibitors and calcium channel blockers. A single agent is often sufficient, but patients may require multiple drugs aimed at different pathophysiologic mechanisms. Such synergistic therapy is often more effective than higher doses of a single drug.

If a secondary form of hypertension exists, more specific therapy might be indicated. Adrenal adenomas which overproduce either aldosterone or cortisol require adrenalectomy as does pheochromocytoma. If hyperaldosteronism is a consequence of bilateral adrenal hyperplasia, chronic medical therapy with spironolactone or amiloride is the treatment of choice. Renal artery stenosis can be treated medically but multiple drugs are usually required. Corrective bypass surgery or percutaneous transluminal balloon dilation can cure the hypertension in about 40% of cases. Success depends upon the type of arterial lesion (fibromuscular vs. atherosclerotic), location within the artery, number of stenoses and co-morbid conditions.

Suggested Readings

Blaustein M, Hamlyn JM. Role of natriuretic factor in essential hypertension: a hypothesis. Ann Intern Med 1983;98:785–791.

Guyton AC. Long term regulation of mean arterial pressure: the renal-body fluid pressure control system. In: Guyton AC, ed. Textbook of medical physiology. Philadelphia: W.B. Saunders Co., 1981:259–273.

Kaplan NM. Hypertension: prevalence, risks, and effect of therapy. Ann Intern Med 1983;98:705–709.

Oparil S. Arterial hypertension. In: Wyngaarden JB, Smith LH, eds. Cecil textbook of medicine. 18th ed. Philadelphia: W.B. Saunders Co., 1988;276–293.

Rose BD. Pathogenesis of essential hypertension. In: Rose BD, ed. Pathophysiology of renal disease. New York: McGraw-Hill Book Co., 1987:469–496.

Task Force on Blood Pressure Control in Children. Report of the second task force on blood pressure control in children. Pediatrics 1987;79:1–25.

The 1988 Report of the Joint National Committee on Detection, Evaluation and Treatment of High Blood Pressure. Arch Intern Med 1988;148:1023–1038.

HYPERTENSION PROBLEMS

1. A 20-year-old woman comes to the college infirmary because of an earache, fever and headache, which have been present for 3 days. Three weeks before she had a severe sore throat that lasted 4 days. When she awoke that morning she had puffy eyes. Presently her physical exam shows purulent otitis media, blood pressure 160/112 mm Hg and trace edema of her hands and feet.

   A. You might order all of the tests below. Which **THREE** would you list as most important in your initial evaluation:

      a. Scr
      b. Serum Na^+, K^+, Cl^-, and HCO_3^- concentration
      c. Complete blood count
      d. Urinalysis
      e. Urine culture
      f. Throat culture for streptococcus
      g. Serum complement concentration
      h. Serum albumin concentration
      i. Electrocardiogram

   B. She is hospitalized. Your initial management of her blood pressure should include (Choose **TWO**):

      a. A diuretic
      b. A low protein diet
      c. A low Na^+ diet
      d. A sedative
      e. An angiotensin converting enzyme inhibitor

2. A 59-year-old man is referred by an insurance company for com-

plete examination. You learn that he has been aware of hypertension for about 10 years and has taken a β-blocker with good control for that time. He has a chronic cough related to his habit of cigarette smoking, and frequent headaches.

The physical examination reveals blood pressure 185/120 mm Hg, pulse 80/minute. His fundi have arteriovenous crossing changes, but no hemorrhages or papilledema. The carotids have faint bruits. The heart has an S4 gallop. The lungs are clear. The abdomen is obese. The femoral arteries have faint bruits. The extremities are normal, except for reduced pulses below the knees. Laboratory testing reveals: serum concentrations of Na^+ 142 mEq/L, K^+ 3.4 mEq/L, HCO_3^- 29 mEq/L, creatinine 1.3 mg/dl and glucose 110 mg/dl. Urinalysis: trace protein, no cells, no casts.

A. **Two** diagnostic possibilities include:
   a. Acute glomerulonephritis
   b. Coarctation of the aorta
   c. Primary aldosteronism
   d. Renal artery stenosis
   e. Pheochromocytoma
B. What **one** laboratory test would be most specific as a discriminator:
   a. Serum uric acid concentration
   b. Plasma renin concentration
   c. Plasma aldosterone concentration
   d. Plasma epinephrine concentration
   e. Serum complement concentration
3. Renin has the following actions (choose **ALL** that are correct):
   a. Raises blood pressure by a direct arteriolar constriction
   b. Directly promotes renal tubular Na^+ reabsorption
   c. Catalyzes production of angiotensin I
   d. Promotes renal water reabsorption
   e. Stimulates aldosterone secretion through adrenal renin receptors
4. All of the following directly stimulate renal Na^+ retention **EXCEPT** (Choose **one**):
   a. Norepinephrine
   b. Aldosterone
   c. Angiotensin II
   d. Renin
   e. Cortisol

5. In a 38-year-old man with essential hypertension and a hyperkinetic circulation, increased adrenergic activity would lead to which of the following (Choose **ALL** that are correct):
   a. Increased renin production
   b. Decreased renin production
   c. Increased cardiac output
   d. Decreased cardiac output
   e. Increased PVR
   f. Decreased PVR

6. Use of which of the following drugs might cause an elevation of blood pressure (Choose **ALL** that are correct)?
   a. Ibuprofen (e.g. Advil, Motrin, Nuprin), a NSAID
   b. Nasal decongestants
   c. Nitroglycerin
   d. Prednisone
   e. Insulin

7. Match each patient in Column A with a likely diagnosis from Column B.

Column A
1. A 22-year-old woman with a blood pressure of 180/110 mm Hg and a flank bruit
2. A 45-year-old obese woman with a blood pressure of 180/105 mm Hg, bruises, serum concentrations of glucose 195 mg/dl, Na$^+$ 144 mEq/L and K$^+$ 3.2 mEq/L
3. A 65-year-old man with a history of two myocardial infarctions, blood pressure of 190/120 mm Hg, carotid bruits, urinalysis showing 1+ protein, serum concentrations of creatinine 2.2 mg/dl, Na$^+$ 139 mEq/L and K$^+$ 3.5 mEq/L

Column B
a. Primary aldosteronism
b. Essential hypertension
c. Polycystic kidney disease
d. Atherosclerotic renal artery stenosis
e. Fibromuscular dysplasia of renal arteries
f. Cushing's disease

4. A 50-year-old woman with blood pressure of 180/110 mm Hg, an abdominal mass, serum concentrations of creatinine 2.0 mg/dl, Na^+ 143 and K^+ 4.6 mEq/L and a urinalysis showing microscopic hematuria

5. A 60-year-old woman with blood pressure 180/110 mm Hg, normal physical exam, serum concentrations of creatinine 1.2 mg/dl, Na^+ 145 mEq/L and K^+ 3.0, normal urinalysis

6. A 48-year-old obese woman with blood pressure of 165/105 mm Hg, normal physical exam, serum concentrations of glucose 100 mg/dl, creatinine 1.2 mg/dl, Na^+ 141 mEq/L, K^+ 4.1 mEq/L, and a normal urinalysis

8. A 45-year-old man who has had serial blood pressure measurements of 150/90 mm Hg for the past 6 months consents to physiologic studies for research purposes prior to treatment. He is stabilized on a 200 mEq Na^+ diet for 3 days prior to provocative testing. He remains on this diet throughout the study period.

	24-Hour urinary Na^+	Plasma Volume	Plasma Catecholamines	Plasma Renin	BP
Baseline measurements	200 mEq	3400 ml	500 pg/ml	2 ng/ml/hr	150/90 mm Hg

Match the following pharmacologic maneuvers in Column A with subsequently measured parameters in Column B.

Column A

1. **One day after** one dose of a short-acting powerful diuretic drug
2. During administration of a direct arteriolar vasodilator drug
3. During administration of an adrenergic blocking drug-acting in the central nervous system
4. During administration of an adrenergic agonist, like norepinephrine
5. During administration of cortisol

Column B

	24-Hour urinary Na^+(mEq)	Plasma Volume (ml)	Plasma Catecholamines (pg/ml)	Plasma Renin (ng/ml/hr)	BP (mm Hg)
a.	200	3400	300	1.5	140/85
b.	50	2900	800	5	140/85
c.	100	3800	800	5	140/85
d.	200	3400	800	5	155/95
e.	100	3800	300	1.5	155/95

9. A 28-year-old woman presents with headaches and light-headedness. She denies palpitations, blushing, diaphoresis. She uses no medications which raise blood pressure. There is no family history of hypertension. The physical examination reveals a blood pressure of 174/114 mm Hg in both arms and in one leg. A lower abdominal bruit radiating to the left flank is present. She has no pedal edema, but her rings fit very tightly which, she acknowledges, is a recent change. Laboratory data are urinalysis normal and serum concentrations of glucose 100 mg/dl, creatinine 1.1 mg/dl, Na^+ 140 mEq/L, K^+ 3.6 mEq/L, Cl^- 102 mEq/L, HCO_3^- 25 mEq/L, hemoglobin 15 gm/dl and hematocrit 45%.

You suspect renal artery stenosis as the cause of her hypertension. An arteriogram reveals three concentric 90–95% stenoses along the length of the left renal artery and a slight reduction in left renal size. The right renal artery appears normal and patent and the right kidney is slightly enlarged.

A. Likely pathophysiologic mechanisms at work include (Choose **ALL** that apply):
   a. Elevated production of renin substrate
   b. Elevated production of angiotensin II
   c. Na^+ retention
   d. Arteriolar constriction
   e. Increased myocardial contractility
   f. Increased circulating catecholamines
B. Choose the correct words in the parentheses in sentences 1 and 2:
   1. Left ureteral urine Na^+ concentration is (higher than, lower than, the same as) right ureteral urine Na^+ concentration.
   2. Left renal vein renin concentration is (higher than, lower than, the same as) right renal vein renin concentration.

Answers

Chapter 1—Review of Normal Renal Physiology

1. A. 7.20 B. 7.46 C. 7.27
2. 1. c 2. a 3. b 4. d Tubules reabsorb myoglobin. 5. d
3. A. mg creatinine in specimen = 1400 ml × 70 mg/dl ÷ 100 ml/dl = 980 mg

   B. $$Ccr = \frac{\text{Creatinine excreted/day}}{\text{Scr}} = \frac{980 \text{ mg/day}}{15 \text{mg/L}} = 65 \text{ L/day}$$

   C. 65 L/day ÷ 1.44 = 45 ml/min
   [Actually 65 L/day × 1000 ml/L ÷ (24 hours/day × 60 min/hour)]

   D. No. Creatinine content is too low. Creatinine production of a large muscular man should be close to or above normal adult range of 1–1.5 gm/day. Also formula would predict creatinine

   $$\text{production/day} = \frac{(140 - \text{age}) \times \text{Body wt}}{5}$$
   $$= \frac{120 \times 200 \text{ lbs} \div 2.2 \text{ lb/kg}}{5}$$
   $$= 2182 \text{ mg/day}$$

4. A. $$Ccr = \frac{\text{Creatinine excreted/day}}{\text{Scr}} =$$
   $$\frac{400 \text{ mg/12 hours} \times 24 \text{ hours/day}}{8 \text{ mg/L}} = 100 \text{ L/day}$$
   100 L/day ÷ 1.44 = 69 ml/min

   B. 69 ml/min ÷ 1 M² × 1.73 M² = 120 ml/min (corrected)
   This is normal.

5. a.
6. A. The BUN/Scr ratio of 30 is high. The stable BUN with the increased urea excretion indicates a high urea production. Therefore, possible causes are gastrointestinal bleeding, high protein meals, corticosteroids and tetracycline.

   B. Urea production is normal. Therefore, disproportionally high

BUN is caused by high tubular reabsorption of urea. Possible causes are volume depletion and urinary outflow obstruction.

7. A. 60 L   B. 20 L   C. 5 L
   D. Total body osmoles will be dissolved in 3L more water than before. Therefore new plasma osmolality = 280 mOsm/kg $\times$ 60 kg $\div$ (60 + 3) kg = 267 mOsm/kg
   E. Serum Na^+ concentration would fall proportionately = 140 mEq/L $\times$ 60 kg $\div$ 63 kg = 133 mEq/L

8. 1. b   2. a   3. c   4. b

9. HCO_3^-–decrease; Na^+-decrease; H_2O-decrease

10. A. 1100 ml/day   B. 1.1 kg/day
    C. Total body osmoles will be dissolved in 2.2 kg less water than before the fast. Plasma osmolality after two days

$$= \frac{\text{Total body water} \times \text{plasma osmolality}}{(60\% \text{ of } 70 \text{ kg}) - 2.2 \text{ kg}}$$

$$= \frac{42 \text{ kg} \times 285 \text{ mOsm/kg}}{39.8 \text{ kg}}$$

$$= 301 \text{ mOsm/kg}$$

    D. $Na^+ < 1$ mEq/day; HCO_3^- - 0 mEq/day; K^+- 10–15 mEq/day
    E. Total body water before fast = 60% of 70 kg = 42 L

10 days' loss of water = 1.1 L $\times$ 10 = 11 L

% loss $\approx$ 11 L/42 L $\approx$ 26%

Total fluid compartment Na^+ before fast is the sum of extra- and intracellular Na^+

Extracellular $Na^+ \approx$ 140 mEq/L $\times$ ⅓ $\times$ 42 L

$\approx$ 1960 mEq

Intracellular $Na^+ \approx$ 12 mEq/L $\times$ ⅔ $\times$ 42 L

$\approx$ 336

Total fluid compartment Na^+ before fast $\approx$ 2296 mEq

10 days' Na^+ loss $\approx$ <10 mEq

% loss $\approx$ <10 mEq/2290 mEq $\approx$ <0.4%

Total body K^+ before fast $\approx$ intracellular K^+

$\approx$ ⅔ $\times$ 42 L $\times$ 150 mEq/L

$\approx$ 4200 mEq

10 days' loss of K^+ = 10–15 mEq $\times$ 10 = 100–150 mEq

% loss = 100 mEq/4200 mEq to 150 mEq/4200 mEq

= 2.4 to 3.6%

11. a. The kidney excretes base as HCO_3^-
12. A. e
    B. GRF in L/day = 100 ml/min × 1.44
                    = 144 L/24 mEq/Lday
       Filtered HCO_3^- = 24 mEq/L × 144 L/day
                    = 3456 mEq
    C. 3456 mEq to reabsorb HCO_3^- + 200 mEq to excrete H^+ load
                    = 3656 mEq
13. d. Urea does not affect tonicity.
14. A. 1. a 2. a 3. a 4. b 5. b
    B. b

Chapter 2—Volume Disorders

1. d
2. b
3. a
4. A. Increased   B. Decreased
5. c
6. b, c, e
7. 700 cc blood
   2800 cc normal saline
   7000 cc D5W
8. A. a
   B. The patient drank water
   C. Normal saline, 2000 cc

	D5W (ml/24 hr)	NS (ml/24 hr)
D. Net extra renal loss from skin and respiratory tract minus water of metabolism?	500	0
renal loss?	500	0
GI loss?	1350	1350

   2.7 L of diarrhea a day containing approximately 80 mEq Na^+/L could be replaced with equal portions of normal saline (Na^+ concentration 154 mEq/L) and D5W.
9. A. e
   B. 1 d   2 a   3 e   4 c   5 b
   C. Urine Na^+ concentration = 3 mEq/L

Third spacing; surreptitious vomiting; laxative abuse; internal bleeding

Urine Na^+ concentration = 50 mEq/L

Diuretics; osmotic diuresis; adrenal insufficiency

10. A. a
    B. a, c
11. a

Chapter 3—Tonicity Disorders

1. 1. d 2. c 3. e 4. a 5. b
2. A. a
   B. c

   In an individual with intact water regulation and such severe hypotonicity urine osmolality should be minimum (i.e. maximally dilute) and C_{H_2O} should be maximum.

   C. $C_{osm} = \dfrac{U_{osm} V}{P_{osm}} = \dfrac{200 \text{ mOsm/kg} \times 700 \text{ ml/4 hr}}{250 \text{ mOsm/kg}}$

   $= 560$ ml/4 hr

   $C_{H_2O} = V - C_{osm} = 700 - 560$ ml/4 hr

   $= 140$ ml/4 hr

   $= 0.58$ ml/min or 0.84 L/day

   D. a
   E. 3% saline

   Desired rise in serum Na^+ concentration = $125 - 120$ mEq/L

   $= 5$ mEq/L

   Total body water = 60% of 62 kg = 37 L

   5 mEq/L $\times$ 37 L = 185 mEq Na^+ needed

   185 mEq Na^+ = X ml 3% saline $\times$ 0.52 mEq Na^+/ml

   ml 3% saline needed = 185 mEq $Na^+ \div$ 0.52 mEq Na^+/ml

   $= 356$ ml

3. A. c
   B. Plasma osmolality. This would distinguish true hyponatremia due to nephrotic syndrome from pseudohyponatremia due to hyperlipidemia.

4. A. Rise   D. Rise
   B. Rise   E. Fall
   C. Fall

5.   A.   Estimated osmolality $= 2[\text{Na}] + \dfrac{\text{BUN}}{2.8} + \dfrac{\text{glucose}}{18}$

$$= 2\,[136] + \dfrac{30}{2.8} + \dfrac{80}{18}$$

$$= 272 + 10.7 + 4.4$$

$$= 287 \text{ mOsm/kg}$$

   B.   Isotonic. Ethylene glycol raises osmolality but does not affect tonicity.

   C.   d

6.   1. c   Urine concentration is normal; bladder capacity is reduced
   2. a   Central DI due to head injury
   3. b   Nephrogenic DI due to chronic interstitial nephritis
   4. d   High fluid intake mimics psychogenic polydipsia

7.   Estimated plasma osmolality $= 2 \times \text{Na}^+$ concentration $= 320$ mOsm/kg

Estimated body water $= 60\%$ of body weight $= \dfrac{22 \text{ lb} \times .6}{2.2 \text{ lb/kg}} = 6 \text{ kg}$

Total body osmoles $= 6 \text{ kg} \times 320 \text{ mOsm/kg} = 1920 \text{ mOsm}$
Assume normal osmolality $\times$ normal body water $=$ current body osmoles

$$285 \text{ mOsm/kg} \times \text{X kg} = 1920 \text{ mOsm}$$

Normal body water or $\text{X} = \dfrac{1920 \text{ mOsm}}{285 \text{ mOsm/kg}} = 6.7 \text{ kg}$

Water deficit $= 6.7 \text{ kg} - 6 \text{ kg} = 0.7 \text{ kg or L}$

8.   a, c. Weight loss would be useful in determining the degree of fluid loss. Urine specific gravity would show if the urine is appropriately concentrated in response to hypertonicity. If a low specific gravity is found, a defect in urine concentration (such as nephrogenic or central diabetes insipidus) would probably account for the hypertonic state. Ethanol as a cause of the hypertonicity is not a consideration since the elevated Na^+ concentration easily accounts for the rise in plasma osmolality. The water deprivation test is used to increase plasma osmolality above the normal range in order to stimulate ADH release. Plasma osmolality is already elevated in this patient.

Chapter 4—Acid-Base Disorders

1. A. b
   B. a. Since the anion gap is not increased, possible etiologies include, in theory, all those listed as causing normal anion gap acidosis, in Table 4.1. However, in view of the failure to maximally acidify the urine and hypokalemia, it is most likely that one is dealing with renal tubular acidosis. This is probably renal tubular acidosis, proximal variety, in which a defect in reabsorption of filtered HCO_3^- exists. At low plasma HCO_3^- levels, the urine may be acid in this condition, but as soon as the plasma concentration of HCO_3^- is increased beyond the tubular capacity for reabsorption urine pH rises and the urine contains large amounts of HCO_3^-. Accompanying disorders may include glycosuria, hyperuricosuria, hypouricemia, aminoaciduria, hyperphosphaturia and hypophosphatemia (Fanconi's syndrome)

2. A. c, d. A high plasma HCO_3^- concentration could result either from respiratory acidosis or metabolic alkalosis.
   B. c. A plasma pH or pCO_2 would distinguish these two possibilities and would define the acid-base disorder.

3. A. Na_2SO_4, CO_2, H_2O
   B. 43 mEq, 42 mEq by HCO_3^- and 1 mEq by protein
   C. Na^+ 140 mEq/L, Cl^- 104 mEq/L, HCO_3^- 20 mEq/L
      The 42 mEq H_2SO_4 consumes 42 mEq HCO_3^-; the HCO_3^- concentration falls by 42 mEq ÷ 10 L or 4.2 mEq/L
   D. Old anion gap $= [Na^+] - ([Cl^-] + [HCO_3^-])$
      $$= 140 - (104 + 24)\ mEq/L$$
      $$= 12\ mEq/L$$
      New anion gap $= 16\ mEq/L$
      Change in anion gap $= 16 - 12\ mEq/L$
      $$= +4\ mEq/L$$

4. A. 32 nEq/L
   B. 7.48
   C. d. The patient has a metabolic alkalosis with a high urine Cl^- concentration. This is usually due to increased mineralocorticoid activity such as seen in primary aldosteronism.
   D. The dramatic fall in urine Cl^- concentration would be observed with the cessation of diuretics.

5. 1. e   2. e   3. c   4. b   5. a
6. A. pH = 7.1
   B. d
   C. Acute, $\Delta HCO_3^- = 0.1 \, \Delta pCO_2$
7. A. a
   B. Lactic acidosis
   C. He is hyperventilating to compensate for the metabolic acidosis
   D. a, d
   E. b, d. Blood pressure must be corrected with adequate blood replacement and $NaHCO_3$ must be given to raise HCO_3^- concentration to 10 mEq/L. The amount needed is 50% of body weight $\times \Delta [HCO_3^-] = 35L \times 7$ mEq/L = 245 mEq.
8. A. Respiratory alkalosis and metabolic acidosis with a normal anion gap. The abnormal HCO_3^- concentration and pCO_2 indicate an acid-base disturbance. Since no primary disorder undergoes complete correction, the normal pH in this patient tells us that he has a combined alteration. Acetazolamide causes metabolic acidosis. Salicylates stimulate ventilation and produce respiratory alkalosis.
   B. Metabolic acidosis with an elevated anion gap. The fall in pCO_2 of 15 mEq/L from normal is 1.3 times the fall in HCO_3^- concentration from normal, which shows the expected respiratory compensation for metabolic acidosis.
   C. c. At this stage of salicylate poisoning unknown acid(s) are produced. In the buffering process these acids react with and "consume" HCO_3^- so that the administered $NaHCO_3$ has no effect on the serum HCO_3^- concentration.
9. A. Respiratory acidosis caused by lung disease and pulmonary edema.
   B. Worsening of respiratory acidosis. The rise in HCO_3^- concentration to 40 mEq/L is a ΔHCO_3^- of 16 mEq/L. This change is $0.4 \times \Delta pCO_2$ so that it is an appropriate renal compensation for chronic respiratory acidosis.
   C. Posthypercapneic metabolic alkalosis
   D. Chloride must be provided. Usually NaCl and KCl are given, but if hypervolemia and hyperkalemia are present NH_4Cl, HCl or arginine HCl may be given.
10. H^+ concentration = 24 nEq/L.
    Metabolic alkalosis with the appropriate respiratory compensa-

tion would explain the acid-base disorder, but not the anion gap of 27 mEq/L. The clinical setting leads one to suspect a metabolic acidosis with an elevated anion gap due to renal failure superimposed on metabolic alkalosis due to nasogastric suction resulting in an alkalemia.

Therapeutic modalities include administration of histaminic H_2 receptor blocking drugs to reduce gastric acid secretion, dialysis against a special low HCO_3^- high Cl^- bath to reduce the HCO_3^- concentration and, rarely, administration of HCl intravenously (as HCl/or arginine hydrochloride). Administration of K^+ has a limited role because the serum K^+ is normal and the patient is oliguric (see chapter on K^+ disorders).

11. A. Metabolic acidosis with an elevated anion gap due to lactic acidosis.
    B. Same acid-base disorder, but the administration of concentrated $NaHCO_3^-$ solution has improved pH and caused hypernatremia.
    C. Metabolic alkalosis. The elevated anion gap is now normal, because the lactate has been metabolized to HCO_3^-. When this regenerated HCO_3^- is added to the administered HCO_3^- an excessive concentration results. This is called "overshoot alkalosis" since it is caused by excessive HCO_3^- administration.

12. A. Metabolic acidosis and respiratory acidosis. The appropriate respiratory compensation for metabolic acidosis would reduce pCO_2 below the normal range. The failure to do this is evidence of respiratory acidosis due to respiratory insufficiency.
    B. Mechanical ventilation could lower pCO_2 to its appropriate level of compensation $\backsim$20 mm Hg, which would halve H^+ to 60 nEq/L (pH = 7.22).

Chapter 5—Potassium Disorders

1. A. b, c. In view of the acidosis, the cause of the hypokalemia could either be renal tubular acidosis (RTA) or chronic loss of alkaline intestinal secretions. The acid urine pH would be consistent with either proximal RTA or diarrhea.
   B. c. If the loss of the potassium is through the gastrointestinal tract, the urinary potassium excretion should be low (<25 mEq/day). If the loss of potassium is renal (RTA), the urinary potassium excretion should be high (>25 mEq/day).

C. b. If NaHCO₃ were administered to a patient with chronic diarrhea and acidosis, H^+ would shift out of cells in exchange for K^+ which would move into cells, thus lowering plasma K^+.

2. A. a, b. The disorders which cause chronic hypokalemia and metabolic alkalosis include diuretics, vomiting, and mineralocorticoid excess. Patients with primary mineralocorticoid excess tend to be hypertensive so this cause is unlikely. Wrestlers frequently take extreme measures to "get down to weight" for competition, so surreptitious vomiting or use of diuretics are the likely etiologies.

B. a. The urine Cl^- will help distinguish vomiting (will be low), diuretics (will be high or low) and mineralocorticoid excess (will be high).

3. A. b. In diabetic ketoacidosis osmotic diuresis increases urine flow and induces volume depletion and hyperaldosteronism. Also the nonreabsorbable acid anions, acetoacetate and β-hydroxybutyrate are presented to the distal nephron. Hence, urinary potassium excretion is enhanced and body potassium stores are reduced.

B. a, b, c. Since diabetic ketoacidosis is a catabolic state, tissues are broken down and intracellular K^+ is released. At the same time the distribution of potassium between the intra- and extracellular compartments is altered by the insulin deficiency and hyperglycemia, resulting in hyperkalemia in the face of reduced body potassium stores.

C. a, b, c, d. Correction of hyperglycemia and catabolic state with insulin alters the distribution of potassium between the intra- and extracellular compartments such that K^+ enters cells and, in the face of reduced body K^+ stores, plasma K^+ plummets to very low levels. Also, the plasma HCO_3^- is high due to over-zealous NaHCO₃ administration and metabolism of the acid anions, acetoacetate and β-hydroxybutyrate, which results in the regeneration of HCO_3^-. This factor also tends to drive K^+ into cells in exchange for H^+.

4. A. b. He has shock and resultant tissue ischemia with lactic acidosis and potassium release from ischemic tissues, especially the right leg. The lactic acidosis per se has not caused the hyperkalemia. Oliguria does not play a role in the development of hyperkalemia in the acute setting.

B. b. If the electrocardiogram is normal attempts should be made to 1) shift potassium into the intracellular space (e.g. with administration of glucose and insulin, and $NaHCO_3$) and 2) restore tissue perfusion (hence, reducing release of K^+ from ischemic tissue), if possible. In all patients with hyperkalemia, serum K^+ and the EKG should be monitored closely.

C. e. He remains in shock and the right lower extremity is necrosing; large amounts of K^+ are now being released from the muscles in the extremity, a rich source of potassium. The ratio of intra- to extracellular K^+ is so altered that there are life-threatening EKG changes. Intravenous Ca^{2+} should be administered immediately to restore cardiac electrophysiology toward normal. Attempts to shift K^+ into cells should also continue, and in addition efforts to remove K^+ from the body (e.g. dialysis, Kayexalate) are mandatory.

Chapter 6—Glomerular Disorders

1. 1. g 2. c 3. a 4. b 5. d 6. h 7. f 8. i 9. e
2. A. d. Hypervolemia is seen with heart failure or the nephritic syndrome, but not with lipoid nephrosis.
   B. c. The impetiginous rash suggests poststreptococcal GN.
3. 1. a (severe crescentic GN)
   2. f (poststreptococcal GN)
   3. d (Henoch-Schonlein purpura)
   4. g (bacterial endocarditis)
   5. c (Goodpasture's syndrome)
   6. b (Alport's syndrome)
   7. e (chronic GN)
4. A. c B. a
5. b. Low complement levels suggest lupus nephritis or subacute bacterial endocarditis. The absent murmur and splenomegaly make endocarditis less likely.
6. A. e. Berger's disease rarely causes a full nephritic syndrome with edema.
   B. d. Physical examination excludes hypervolemia; normal fundi exclude diabetic nephropathy. The draining sinus suggests the possibility of amyloidosis due to a chronic inflammatory process.

7. a. Normal serum albumin excludes nephrotic syndrome. Hypervolemia is not present on physical examination.
8. 1. b   2. c   3. f   4. e   5. d   or b   6. a   7. g
9. 1. g   2. f   3. e   4. a   5. d   6. b   7. c
10. 1. e   2. f   3. g   4. h

Chapter 7—Renal Perfusion Disorders

1. c
2. b, d
3. 1. d   2. a   3. b   4. c
4. b, c
5. c. The clinical setting and the history are very suggestive of left renal artery embolism.
6. d. This patient has developed hepatorenal syndrome.
7. b

Chapter 8—Disorders of Urinary Outflow

1. e   6. b
2. b   7. b
3. d   8. a
4. e   9. e
5. b   10. c

Chapter 9—Acute Renal Failure

	Other Helpful Physical Findings	Urinalysis	Laboratory	Clinical Course	Diagnosis
Case 1	c	e	a	a	a
Case 2	e	b	c	e	e
Case 3	f	a	f	f	d
Case 4	a	c	e	c	b
Case 5	d	f	b	b	c
Cast 6	b	d	d	d	f

Chapter 10—Chronic Renal Failure

1. A. Fall   E. Either   H. Rise
   B. Rise   F. Fall   I. Rise
   C. Fall   G. Rise   J. Either
   D. Fall
2. A. a, d
   B. c
3. b
4. 1. g 2. c 3. c 4. e 5. a 6. a, b 7. d 8. f

Chapter 11—Urinalysis

1. A. No. Why? 3+ proteinuria and red cell casts point to a renal source
   B. Membranoproliferative GN. Gross hematuria, red cell casts and 3+ proteinuria suggest both a nephritic and nephrotic picture. Since the clinical picture does not fit lupus nephritis, membranoproliferative is the most likely diagnosis. Acute proliferative GN and IgA nephropathy are also possibilities.
2. Proximal RTA. RTA is diagnosed by failure of urine to acidify <5.5 in patients with acidemia. Glycosuria suggests Fanconi's syndrome.
3. No. Why? There are no red cells in the urine.
4. ATN. Isotonic urine in a hypotensive patient and brown granular casts exclude prerenal azotemia.
5. Diabetes mellitus with osmotic diuresis due to glycosuria.
6. No. Why? No WBCs or bacteria.
7. Repeat urinalysis after avoiding exercise. Why? Amber color—normal in concentrated urine. Protein—may be normal in urine this concentrated (150 mg protein/500 ml = 30 mg/dl = 1+). Ketones—due to fasting. Few red cells—may be seen after exercise. Amorphous urates—may be seen normally in concentrated or cool specimen. Sperm—normal finding.

Chapter 12—Hypertension

1. A. a, d and f
   B. a, c

Her collection of symptoms suggests an acute bacterial infection. Suspicion for streptococcus should be high and her history of a prior pharnygitis arouses further suspicion. She has physical evidence for Na^+ retention in edema and moderate hypertension. Acute poststreptococcal glomerulonephritis is the leading diagnostic possibility. Initial tests should evaluate for this. A diuretic and low Na^+ diet attack hypervolemia, the presumed mechanism of her hypertension most directly.

2. A. c, d
    B. b
    This man has longstanding hypertension which is escaping control. He has physical evidence for diffuse atherosclerosis. You should suspect renal artery stenosis as a secondary cause, superimposed upon what probably has been essential hypertension. The hypokalemia is biochemical evidence for high aldosterone activity. This is consistent with renal artery stenosis *or* primary hyperaldosteronism, which is reasonable. The best discriminator would be a plasma renin assay. It should be high with renal artery stenosis and low with primary aldosteronism.

3. c
Renin is an enzyme which catalyzed production of angiotensin I from renin substrate (angiotensinogen). It has no direct tubular, arteriolar or adrenal actions.

4. d
Renin has no direct tubular action.

5. a, c, and e
See text and Figure 12.2.

6. a, b and d
Nonsteroidal anti-inflammatory drugs promote Na^+ and H_2O retention and inhibit vasodilator prostaglandin actions. Most nasal decongestants are sympathomimetic. Prednisone is a widely prescribed cortisol analogue used as an anti-inflammatory agent.

7. 1. e
    2. f
    3. d
    4. c
    5. a
    6. b

8. 1. b

2. c
3. a
4. d
5. e

Following administration of a diuretic, plasma volume is contracted; therefore, the kidney retains Na^+ and catecholamine and renin levels will rise.

A direct arteriolar vasodilator lowers blood pressure; therefore, the kidney retains Na^+ and plasma catecholamine and renin levels reflexly rise. Plasma volume increases as a result of Na^+ retention.

A centrally acting adrenergic blocker will lower blood pressure by lowering renin output and catecholamine levels. Plasma volume and Na^+ balance are not significantly affected at first, since lower blood pressure reduces filtered Na^+, but lower catecholamine levels reduce tubular Na^+ reabsorption.

Of course, an adrenergic agonist (stimulant) will raise blood pressure, plasma catecholamines and renin. Plasma volume and Na^+ excretion are not initially affected.

Cortisol causes retention of Na^+ and expansion of plasma volume. Blood pressure rises. Catecholamines are slightly lower. Renin output would be mildly suppressed by the hypervolemia.

9. A. b, c and d
    B. a. Lower than
       b. Higher than

Renal artery stenosis produces hypertension through angiotensin II, which causes arteriolar constriction and Na^+ retention. Catecholamines and myocardial function should be reduced.

The stenosed kidney is underperfused while the contralateral kidney is hyperperfused. Thus, the stenosed kidney produces renin but retains Na^+. The hyperperfused contralateral kidney has very little renin production and excretes Na^+. Actually, this physiologic observation is used diagnostically: one hopes to demonstrate high unilateral venous output of renin with contralateral suppression of renin production.

Appendix

Normal Laboratory Values and Conversion Factors from Conventional to SI (Systéme International) Units

Test	Normal Range		Conversion Factor
	Conventional Units	SI Units	
Blood, Serum or Plasma			
Scr	≤1.5 mg/dl	≤133 μmol/L	88.4
BUN	≤20 mg/dl	≤7.1 mmol/L (of urea)	0.357
BUN/Scr ratio	10–15	40–61 (Scr expressed as mmol/L)	4.04
Osmolality	280–290 mOsm/kg	Same	
Na^+	135–145 mEq/L	135–145 mmol/L	1
K^+	3.5–5 mEq/L	3.5–5 mmol/L	1
H^+	38–43 nEq/L	38–43 nmol/L	1
pH (arterial)	7.37–7.42	Same	
Cl^-	95–105 mEq/L	95–105 mmol/L	1
HCO_3^-	22–28 mEq/L	22–28 mmol/L	1
pCO2 (arterial)	37–43 mm Hg	Same	
Albumin	4–5 gm/dl	40–50 g/L	10
Anion gap	8–14 mEq/L	8–14 mmol/L	1
Calcium	8.5–10.5 mg/dl	2.1–2.6 mmol/L	0.25
Phosphate (as phosphorus)	2.5–5.0 mg/dl	0.8–1.6 mmol/L	0.323

Urinalysis			
pH	4.5–8	Same	
Specific gravity	1.001–1.004	Same	
Osmolality	50–1200 mOsm/kg	Same	
Protein	Negative or trace (<1+) (<15 mg/dl)	Same (<150 mg/L)	10
Glucose	negative	Same	
Ketone	negative	Same	
Red cells	<5 rbc/hpf	Same	
White cells	<5 wbc/hpf	Same	
Bacteria	0	Same	Same
Daily Urinary Excretion			
Creatinine	1.0–1.5 gm/day	9–13 mmol/day	8.84
GFR or Ccr	80–120 ml/min (115–173 L/day)	1.33–2.00 ml/s	0.0167
Protein	<150 mg/day	0.150 gm/day	0.001
Water (average)	0.5–12L	Same	
	1.5L	Same	
Na$^+$ (average)	150 mEq/day	150 mmol/day	1
K$^+$ (average)	60–120 mEq/day	60–120 mmol/day	1
H$^+$ (average)	70–100 nEq/day	70–120 nmol/day	1
Osmoles (average)	600 mOsm/day	Same	1

Index

Page numbers in *italics* denote figures; those followed by "t" denote tables.